CRISIS
INTERVENTION

Scott Fraser provides kind, encouraging, and inspiring insight into the challenges of both psychotherapy and the essence of crisis intervention. Dr. Fraser's relatable book is highly readable and practical. It is an evidence-based yet efficient approach to treatment. The book is a new, more efficient approach to professional assistance. It's both helpful systematically and in practice guidelines, such as his process of change model. Highly recommended.

—**Charles R. Figley, PhD**, Kurzweg Chair in Disaster Mental Health and School of Social Work, Tulane University, New Orleans, LA

Drawing on his extensive experience, Scott Fraser rewards us with an innovative and far-reaching orientation to crisis. Fraser poses a striking challenge to common sense responses to crises and provides rich illustrations of his counter-intuitive view in action. A useful and deeply engaging work.

—**Kenneth J. Gergen, PhD**, Swarthmore College, Swarthmore, PA

In his highly innovative volume, J. Scott Fraser offers a fresh, process-based approach to crisis intervention. His focus on tipping points, those critical moments of decision and change, aligns closely with what we know about the role of context, flexibility, and values in creating long-lasting change. This book invites practitioners to step into the dynamic flow of crises, not just to resolve them, but to use them as catalysts for growth. Fraser's work speaks to anyone willing to see crises as precious windows of opportunity and is a necessary read for practitioners wishing to deepen their work when everything is on the line.

—**Steven C. Hayes, PhD**, Foundation Professor Emeritus, University of Nevada, Reno, and originator of acceptance and commitment therapy (ACT)

The tipping point interventions and the process of change model presented in this book are inspiring ways to work with people in crisis situations for optimal outcomes. This book is a must-read for professionals who work with clients in crisis situations and want a new way forward.

—**Toni Zimmerman, PhD, LMFT**, Professor, Human Development and Family Studies Department, and Program Director for the Marriage and Family Therapy Graduate Program, Colorado State University, Fort Collins

Scott Fraser's *Crisis Intervention* fills a much-needed gap in the psychotherapy literature. Much of that work is grounded in the presumption that clinicians must slowly and methodically assess and plan, yet much of clinical practice requires great urgency. Fraser offers a new vision of how to proceed in the context of crisis, centered in an overarching process of change model that includes a systemic vision that extends beyond the individual, and a view in which crisis is not equated with disaster but as presenting opportunities for fundamental change. Well written and filled with illustrative examples, the book is authored by a skillful clinician who has worked for years in this context. I highly recommend this book to all practicing mental health professionals, and this should be essential reading for all students in training to be psychotherapists.

—**Jay Lebow, PhD**, Clinical Professor and Senior Scholar, The Family Institute at Northwestern and Northwestern University, Evanston, IL

This book masterfully extends the seminal Mental Research Institute brief therapy model to the arena of crisis intervention. Drawing on systemic and social constructivist ideas, Scott Fraser shows how crises such as trauma, suicidality, grief, domestic violence, and sexual assault present windows of opportunity for clinicians to tip vicious cycles of problem maintenance in new and positive directions through strategic, often counterintuitive intervention.

—**Michael J. Rohrbaugh, PhD**, Professor Emeritus of Psychology, University of Arizona, Tucson

CRISIS
INTERVENTION

Using Tipping Points to Achieve
Transformative Change in Therapy

J. Scott Fraser

 AMERICAN PSYCHOLOGICAL ASSOCIATION

Published by
American Psychological Association
750 First Street, NE
Washington, DC 20002
https://www.apa.org

Order Department
https://www.apa.org/pubs/books
order@apa.org

Typeset in Charter and Interstate by Circle Graphics, Inc., Reisterstown, MD

Printer: Sheridan Books, Chelsea, MI
Cover Designer: Gwen J. Grafft, Minneapolis, MN

Library of Congress Cataloging-in-Publication Data
Names: Fraser, J. Scott, author.
Title: Crisis intervention : using tipping points to achieve transformative
   change in therapy / by J. Scott Fraser.
Description: Washington, DC : American Psychological Association, [2025] |
   Includes bibliographical references and index.
Identifiers: LCCN 2024031745 (print) | LCCN 2024031746 (ebook) | ISBN
   9781433843341 (paperback) | ISBN 9781433843358 (ebook)
Subjects: LCSH: Psychotherapy. | Crisis intervention (Mental health
   services)
Classification: LCC RC480.6 .F75 2025 (print) | LCC RC480.6 (ebook) | DDC
   616.89/025—dc23/eng/20240828
LC record available at https://lccn.loc.gov/2024031745
LC ebook record available at https://lccn.loc.gov/2024031746

https://doi.org/10.1037/0000445-000

Contents

Preface   *vii*

Acknowledgments   *ix*

Introduction: Tipping Point Interventions and the Process
of Change   3

I. CRISIS, CHAOS, CATASTROPHE, AND THE PROCESS
OF CHANGE   11

1. Traditional Crisis Intervention and Its Problems   15

2. The Theory Base for the Process of Change Model in Crisis
   Intervention and Brief Therapy   21

3. Viewing Crises Through the Process of Change   41

4. Doing Crisis Intervention From the Process View   55

II. TIPPING POINT INTERVENTIONS ACROSS CRISES:
FOLLOWING THE PROCESS OF CHANGE MODEL   75

5. Trauma: Stress, Disorder, and Growth   79

6. Suicidal Crises: Hazardous Intersections   105

7. Grief and Mourning   131

8. Intimate Partner Violence: Time-Limited Windows
   of Opportunity   157

9. Sexual Assault: Intervening in Culturally Shaped Crises   185

10. Tipping Points and Windows of Opportunity   217

References   *231*
Index   *251*
About the Author   *263*

Preface

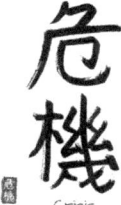
Crisis

The Chinese characters *wei ji* that open this chapter are commonly used to symbolize the term *crisis*. They have been popularized in speeches by political figures like U.S. President John F. Kennedy addressing international crises; by former vice president, Al Gore, in speeches on climate change; and by numerous motivational business speakers on grasping opportunity out of dangerous crises. John F. Kennedy in a speech to the Convocation of the United Negro College Fund on April 12, 1959, and in many speeches thereafter in the run-up to the election in 1960 used the following definition of crisis:

> When written in Chinese, the word "crisis" is composed of two characters—one represents danger and one represents opportunity.

This is a crucial point for us all to remember, as we will discuss in this book. However, the popularization of these crisis characters, while useful in many ways, is technically flawed. In an essay titled, "How a Misunderstanding About Chinese Characters Has Led Many Astray," Victor H. Mair (2009), a professor of Chinese language and literature, noted the following:

> While it is true that wēijī does indeed mean "crisis" and that the wēi syllable of wēijī does convey the notion of "danger," the jī syllable of wēijī most definitely does not signify "opportunity." The jī of wēijī, in fact, means something like "incipient moment," [or a] crucial point (when something begins or changes). . . . Aside from the notion of "incipient moment" or "crucial point" discussed above, the graph for jī by itself indicates "quick-witted(ness); resourceful(ness)." (p. 1)

In this book, we will discuss the idea that what is considered as a crisis differs from one person, group, or context to another. At times, something described as a crisis will be dangerous and require attention to decrease its risks. At other times, it may simply signal potential significant changes. Yet, the latter meanings of the character, ji, as the quality of quick-witted(ness) and resourceful(ness) will most always determine the future successful path for those engaged around a crisis point—both as clients and as practitioners. Crises must be embraced as tipping points for better or worse, depending on what those engaged at those points do to move beyond them. This is the essential message of this book.

The Chinese characters *wei ji* represent the tipping points for all involved in a potential crisis. For clients, *tipping points* are critical choice points in the changing patterns of their life when the way they describe and react to their perceived dilemma may initiate the vicious cycle of a crisis, absorb the dilemma into the normal patterns of their life, or seize the opportunity of the dilemma to initiate new and positive virtuous cycle patterns in their lives and those of others. Similarly, for those involved helping others and practitioners, their intersection with those in potential distress or crisis may be viewed as a *hazardous intersection* to be returned to safe normality, or as a *window of opportunity* where all involved are open to choose what may have been seen as risky, or even counterintuitive, shifts in the past but with support and guidance of an intervenor may open new and fulfilling lifepaths. These are critical choice points for both clients and practitioners. How all involved view and respond to these choice points will most often determine the future direction of their lives. This book will tie together the literature on how successful choices can be embraced across a wide range of different crises to seize opportunities from the potential dangers of crises. It will also trace tipping point interventions as they are linked through the process of change model of crisis intervention and brief therapy.

Acknowledgments

This book is dedicated to the staff of the Crisis/Brief Therapy Center of what was the Good Samaritan Hospital Community Mental Health Center in Dayton, Ohio, and to all the clients in crisis we served over the years in the center, the emergency room, and with the police. I couldn't have had a better set of colleagues who shared support, humor, caring, and high levels of skill with everyone we served. I also want to acknowledge all the doctoral students, "expediters," and trainees who worked and trained in this outstanding unit and who excelled in courses and dissertations through the doctoral program of the Wright State University School of Professional Psychology. Thanks again to Susan Reynolds of APA Books, whose continued faith and support in my work helped make this book possible. Finally, my ongoing gratitude goes to my wife, Beth Fraser, for her love, patience, and support that have sustained me throughout this project and over the years.

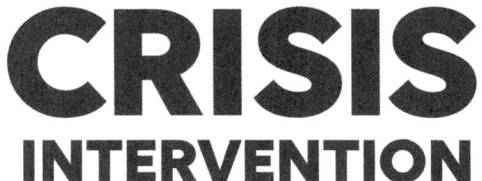

CRISIS
INTERVENTION

INTRODUCTION
Tipping Point Interventions and the Process of Change

This book aims to revise the traditional notion of crisis and how to do crisis intervention and brief therapy. Most practitioners across helping disciplines have been taught to assess danger and reduce risks. This book will explain how to seize the opportunity of crises and tip them toward rapid resolution. It will help readers view crises as time-limited windows of opportunity to move all the people involved in new and positive directions in their lives. It will teach a viewpoint and model for understanding crises in their context, engaging with all involved using their values, culture, and language, honoring their goals, and changing vicious cycles into virtuous ones. It will also show how different types of crises nonetheless reflect similar vicious cycles, and how each of those vicious cycles can be successfully tipped toward resolution by embracing what we refer to as the *process of change model of crisis and crisis intervention*. While this perspective can often seem complex and different from our everyday views of our world, perhaps a few different crisis examples along with their intervention strategies will help.

Consider the following cases: A therapist agrees with his suicidal patient that from his client's view, life does seem hopeless, and he can see why his

https://doi.org/10.1037/0000445-001
Crisis Intervention: Using Tipping Points to Achieve Transformative Change in Therapy, by J. S. Fraser

client wants to die. Another therapist counsels her client after a recent beating by her husband and warns her that leaving is a dangerous moment and should be undertaken with care. Another client trying to recover from a traumatic event is coached to relive that event in detail while writing it down. A grieving spouse returns with her therapist to the favorite place she and her husband would go for breakfast and talks to her therapist about him there. These interventions are counterintuitive in some ways, yet each was successful.

Now contrast those cases with these: Another client died feeling despondent and isolated despite their therapist and family insisting that life was worth living. Another woman, at the urging of her friends, left her husband and was killed by him shortly after leaving. In another instance, a rape survivor continued to have flashbacks of the attack despite her efforts to put it out of her mind. Still another woman found herself grieving years after the death of her partner, despite her efforts to stay busy. These examples represent failures of logical reactions to crises; these responses made sense, yet they made things worse. These two sets of cases are opposites of each other. We will make sense of this in Chapters 1 and 2 of this volume.

As we move forward, we will discuss how people are drawn into a crisis and typically resort to logical, tried-and-true responses to resolve them. Sometimes they do end up resolving them as, by definition, those responses have been useful in the past. However, at other times, those very solutions that have always been helpful only serve to make things worse, as they did in the second set of examples. In the first case examples, these clients reversed their solution patterns around their crises by doing something very different from or even opposite of their former solution patterns and thus began the process of change and resolution.

In the next few chapters, we will see that crises often evolve from what may appear to be a minor shift in the way things have always been—or potential tipping points. Then, depending on how that shift is interpreted and subsequently acted upon, clients may spiral into a vicious cycle, often ending in disaster, continued suffering, or loss of life. And, as in the first seemingly counterintuitive case interventions just described, effective crisis interventions frequently involve stepping out of an initial mindset and typical responses to try powerfully effective yet often paradoxical solutions when seen from the original points of view. Crises may also occur at different levels of systems yet follow the same process.

Consider, for example, the events in Mann Gulch, Montana, in 1949, described next. A disaster evolved from a small, seemingly harmless fire to a major conflagration that threatened smokejumpers' lives, and then to an ingenious solution, which was not followed by others because it was so opposite of what they had always known to do.

> A forest fire which seemed harmless at first was waiting to explode. A team of fifteen smokejumpers parachuted in to contain the fire, but soon they were running for their lives, racing to the top of a steep ridge. Their foreman, Wag Dodge, recognized that they would not make it, and had his men drop their tools and run up the hill.
>
> With the fire barely two hundred yards behind him, he did a strange and marvelous thing. He invented a solution. His crew must have thought he had gone crazy as he took some matches out of his pocket, bent down and set fire to the grass directly in front of him. The fire spread quickly uphill, and he stepped into the middle of the newly burnt area, calling for his crew to run back into his newly set fire and join him in the now burned area behind it which wouldn't burn as the fire would have no fuel and leap over it.
>
> But nobody followed Wag Dodge. They ignored him, clinging to what they had been taught, and they ran right by the answer. The fire raged past Wag Dodge and overtook the crew, killing thirteen men and burning 3,200 acres. Dodge survived, nearly unharmed. (Berwick, 2002, pp. 12–13)

Wag Dodge's solution was counterintuitive from the perspective of his team. As in the first set of cases at the start of this chapter, Dodge's crisis resolution stepped out of the assumptions, definitions, and consequent reactions of how to respond to wildfires at that time. Since then, setting escape fires of the kind Wag Dodge used has become standard procedure for fire jumpers. Eventually another seemingly paradoxical policy change directed firefighters to let many fires to burn instead of putting them all out. The idea is to allow the fires to clear brush that might eventually ignite an even larger fire—in essence allowing forest fires to burn to prevent future forest fires. This was the same process of crisis pattern development, reversal, and resolution as in the first set of cases described earlier in this chapter. As I will explain, the process of crises evolution and resolution is the same across different types of crises, including often counterintuitive pattern shifts from initial vicious cycles.

Now consider this Japanese folktale:

> A Japanese coastal village was once threatened by a tidal wave, but the wave was sighted in advance, far out on the horizon, by a lone farmer in the rice fields on the hillside above the village. At once he set fire to the fields, and the villagers who came swarming up to save their crops were saved from the flood. (de Shazer, 1991; Fraser, 1995a)

Once more, an effective solution to an impending disaster was counterintuitive. In this case, a small trigger of setting a fire on the hill saved the villagers. There was no time to explain the villagers' impending drowning in a tsunami. The farmer on the hill relied on the villagers' interpretation of the crisis as the potential loss of their crops to the fire to draw them up the hill and to safety. The villagers' interpretation of their situation, the way they viewed the potential loss of their crops, triggered their rush up the hill. Running to higher ground saved them from the coming tsunami, yet they took that action for a different purpose. In this folktale, as in all cases, what is viewed as a crisis, and what type of crisis, is based on the culture, language, and traditions of those involved and their context as they see it. In this case, the lone farmer understood the villagers' fear of both losing their crops and losing their lives to drowning in a tsunami. What would have made most sense in this situation would have been for him to run down from the hillside to warn the villagers. Yet there was no time. All would have been drowned in the tsunami, including him. At that tipping point, the farmer instead thought quickly and creatively and took the paradoxical and counterintuitive action of setting the rice fields on fire. His quick, ingenious solution within his cultural context embraced this tipping point and saved the villagers. As we will see, such small and often counterintuitive shifts from what makes sense are often the hallmark of successful crisis resolution.

Similarly, in the classic movie *It's a Wonderful Life* (Capra, 1946), the angel, Clarence Odbody, saved the main character, George Bailey, from jumping off a bridge to kill himself—by himself jumping off that bridge. Just as we will advocate for all crisis intervention practitioners to do, Clarence aligned himself with George's lifelong value of helping others. In doing so, he prevented George from dying by suicide, instead prompting him to jump off the bridge and into the swirling cold water to save Clarence rather than to end his own life.

Each of these examples shows the first key to understanding the process-based view on how crises develop and how they are often resolved. That is, crises are invariably vicious cycle patterns of well-intentioned attempts to solve or ameliorate a perceived challenging situation. Such repeated solutions are shaped by the norms, language, culture, and experiences of what has typically worked and is appropriate. Such solutions are often seen as tried-and-true because they have usually worked in the past. However, when they falter in urgent and potentially risky situations, these rigidly repeated solutions only serve to escalate and exacerbate the ongoing crisis. These crises are often triggered by a relatively minor perceived shift in normal life. The more those involved see risk, danger, and urgency evident in such situations, the more intensely the solutions will be applied and repeated. Doing anything different in such urgent situations is seen as very risky in itself. Yet, as we will see, such counterintuitive actions are quite often the key to crisis resolution. Aligning with the values, worldview, and language and agreeing on goals, new frames, and actions that make sense of the previously counterintuitive solutions is at the core of the process of change model we will advocate in this book. We will have much more to say about aligning with our clients' values and worldviews to help them interdict the vicious cycles of their crises as we discuss the process of change approach to crisis intervention in Chapter 3, but there are a few more perspectives on crises to address first.

CRISES ARE RELATIVE

Crises are always relative to the view of those experiencing them. Some people's crises may be another group's salvation. The following example also shows how one seemingly small event often triggers a cascade of events for better or worse, depending on one's perspective. While this example is still another context for a crisis event and at a larger scale, the same process holds for how virtuous and vicious cycles evolve.

Consider these events: On November 6, 2014, the *New York Times* published an op-ed article with the headline, "How the Fall of the Berlin Wall Really Happened" (Sarotte, 2014). It recounted the events and interactions that led to the opening of the Berlin Wall on the night of November 9, 1989, as a sequence of interchanges that led to cascading events that no one might have ever predicted. Excerpts from this article paint the picture this way:

> In truth, the opening of the Berlin Wall on the night of Nov. 9, 1989, was not planned. Well into that year, East Germany remained nearly inescapable: The last killing by a guard at the wall occurred in February 1989; the last shooting, a very near miss, in April; the last death during an escape attempt on the larger East German border, only 10 days earlier. . . . However, in response to some political climate changes, Politburo members in East Berlin decided to make minor changes to the state's draconian travel rules—but to retain their power to deny travel permission on a whim.
>
> The announcement of this pseudo-reform, at an international news conference televised on the night of Nov. 9, was botched. The bumbling Politburo member running the conference, Günter Schabowski, read the news release for the first time on air. Much of his reading was garbled, but a few phrases popped out: trips abroad would be "possible for every citizen," starting "right away, immediately." Shorn of their context, these phrases mistakenly gave journalists and TV viewers the impression that the wall was open. . . . And so, when tens of thousands of Berliners headed toward the wall in the minutes after the news conference, the entire system cracked.
>
> When one of the regime's most loyal subordinates, a Stasi officer named Harald Jäger who was working the Nov. 9 night shift at a crucial checkpoint in the Berlin Wall, repeatedly phoned his superiors with accurate reports of swelling crowds, they did not trust or believe him. They called him a delusional coward. Insulted, furious and frightened, he decided to let the crowds out, starting a chain reaction that swept across all of the checkpoints that night. (Sarotte, 2014; see also Fraser, 2018, pp. 68–69)

One seemingly random miscommunication produced a cascade of interactions and decisions that spiraled into what turned out to be a historic change of events. From the perspective of the East German government, this was likely seen as a catastrophic crisis or error. From the view of the East German people who wanted to leave, this was their liberation. Whether a pattern is viewed as a vicious or virtuous cycle is always a product of the observer.

CRISES OFTEN RESOLVE BY REFRAMING THEM

Finally, consider the case of John:

> John had gone to the outdoor rock concert with a set of friends, not knowing they had brought along some brownies with marijuana baked into them. His date that day had also brought some sugar cubes with LSD in them. After eating the brownies and a sugar cube, John had to be taken to the concert infirmary. He thought he was going insane. His friends assured him that his reactions were to the drugs and apologized, but the terrible, frightening event continued to play out for John over the next year. Whenever he was in an uncertain situation, or one requiring him to be clearheaded and articulate, he found himself having racing thoughts, a pounding heart, tingling in his hands, and a need to sit down before passing out from hyperventilation. Each time, the more he tried to calm himself down, the more out of control he seemed to become. It wasn't until John went to the university's health service and learned about the physical bases of a panic attack that his troubles went away. (Fraser, 2018, pp. 67–68)

In this case, a classic cascade of successive crises or panic attacks was initiated by one event. The succeeding crises, however, far outlived the drugs originally in John's system that triggered the vicious cycles. His solutions—his hypervigilance and his attempts to calm himself—became the problem. Finally, a relatively minor new bit of information stopped the pattern. John accepted that there was nothing to solve, and by accepting the distress, it went away. This is one more example of the process that inevitably characterizes most all crises. Crises are typically sustained and exacerbated by the solutions aimed at resolving them, and they are most often resolved by simple redirection of those patterns.

THE PLAN OF THIS BOOK

This book is divided into two parts, with Part I laying out the foundation of a process view of change, the evolution of crises, and the process of change model of crisis intervention and brief therapy. Part II traces effective interventions across a range of different crises and drives home how they all fit with the process of change model.

Part I: Crisis, Chaos, Catastrophe, and the Process of Change

The four chapters in Part I address the foundation of a process of change view on crises and crisis intervention. Chapter 1 lays out the problems of the traditional approaches to crisis intervention. Chapter 2 presents the theory and research that are the foundations of the process view. Chapter 3 covers the *viewing* of crises from the process view. Finally, Chapter 4 presents guidelines for the *doing* of crisis intervention from the process of change perspective.

Part II: Tipping Point Interventions Across Crises: Following the Process of Change Model

Part II has six chapters, each covering a different crisis and showing how the process of change links them all in both theory and practice. These chapters cover trauma, suicide, grief and mourning, intimate partner violence, and sexual assault. Chapter 5 on trauma is offered as an overview of what is often encountered across various crises. Chapter 6 on suicide is an example of what we have termed an *incidental crisis*. Chapter 7 on grief and mourning reflects what is mainly a *developmental crisis*, although it is sometimes incidental as in unexpected deaths and killings. Chapters 8 and 9 on intimate partner violence and sexual assault, respectively, are examples of what we have termed *endemic crises* in that they are largely a product of entrenched language and cultural factors. Chapter 10 offers a summary, conclusions, and future directions for practice, applying the process of change model briefly to a range of other crises and addressing the needs of the practitioner before summarizing the model and the take-home messages of the book.

THE PROCESS OF CHANGE MODEL

At the end of each succeeding chapter, a set of bulleted points summarizes the key points of that chapter and moves forward the process of change model of crisis intervention and brief therapy. To initiate that format and to preview the essence of the process of change model, this Introduction concludes with a set of bullet points describing some of the core elements of the model to be laid out in succeeding chapters.

The key elements of the process of change model are as follows:

- Crises evolve from perceived potentially risky shifts in the ongoing flow of peoples' lives.

- Crises are always relative to the norms and views of those experiencing them.

- The form, identity, and process of crises are thus shaped by how such situations are viewed by those involved.

- People will most often use tried-and-true solutions to address these perceived risks.

- When initial solutions fail, rigidly repeated failed solutions feed the vicious cycles of most all crises.

- Shifts in perspectives of the situation and/or shifts in failed solutions are most often the key to crisis resolution.

- However, such shifts from the norm are typically experienced as paradoxical, counterintuitive, and even riskier than the crisis itself.

- Yet people are often most open to new views and solutions when all of their past efforts have repeatedly failed at these tipping points.

- Rapid intervention at such tipping points offers a window of opportunity to introduce often profound redirection of such vicious cycles and even initiate growth and transformation.

- Aligning peoples' values and goals with the new and often creative view and direction often yields not only rapid resolution but also potential growth and transformation.

- Finally, the literature on effective crisis intervention approaches across all different crises follows the same form, thus unifying effective crisis intervention and brief treatment across all crises and models through the process of change model as will be shown in Part II.

PART I CRISIS, CHAOS, CATASTROPHE, AND THE PROCESS OF CHANGE

INTRODUCTION: CRISIS, CHAOS, CATASTROPHE, AND THE PROCESS OF CHANGE

The Chinese Characters for Crisis, Chaos, Catastrophe, and Transformational Change

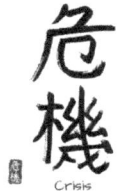

Crisis

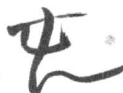 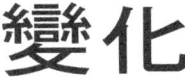

Take a look at the Chinese characters that open this introduction to Part I. As we noted in the Preface, the first set of characters has traditionally been used to symbolize *crisis*. The three characters that follow—*chaos, catastrophe*, and *transformational change*—symbolize the essence of the process of change perspective as it guides crisis intervention. This essence is the focus of Part I of this book and is a foundation for all that follows in Part II.

In Chapters 1 through 4, we will first discuss the concept of *chaos* and how the research on chaos theory informs newer thinking on the process of change. We will note how it helps reshape how we think about the nature of change in our lives and how that influences our choices at crisis points. The character for *catastrophe* represents the now more commonly found process of rapid change that will help us understand how crises may emerge rapidly and resolve just as rapidly with often seemingly small, yet sometimes counterintuitive, shifts in solution patterns around crises. The final Chinese character, *transformational change*, represents the potential in all crisis situations for true transformation in the lives of those involved. This is the promise of embracing tipping points in crises and following the process of change model of intervention that will be explained, illustrated, and followed in Chapter 4 and throughout the chapters in Part II.

1 TRADITIONAL CRISIS INTERVENTION AND ITS PROBLEMS

November 28, 1942, by most accounts, marks the beginning of the organized study of crisis intervention along with a range of other remarkable innovations. The Cocoanut Grove nightclub fire in Boston, Massachusetts, which resulted in 492 deaths, occurred on that date (Schorow, 2005). It was at that time the second-deadliest single-building fire in American history. It was likely caused by a single match lit by a waiter trying to replace a light bulb near the ceiling amidst some flammable artificial palm tree decorations. There were more than 1,000 people celebrating that Thanksgiving weekend during World War II, in a space rated for a maximum of 460. Fire regulations had been ignored: flammable materials had been used in the building, flammable gases were in the air systems, and most exits had been blocked ahead of time to keep out people who had not paid. Hospitals in the Boston area received one casualty every 11 seconds, a historical record (Schorow, 2005).

This disaster was an intense crisis for all involved in the fire and its aftermath. It is also an example of chaos in many ways as well as a positive tipping point in the evolution of medical and psychological responses to all of those in crisis.

https://doi.org/10.1037/0000445-002
Crisis Intervention: Using Tipping Points to Achieve Transformative Change in Therapy, by J. S. Fraser

Briefly, the term *chaos* refers to chaos theory, which describes how open systems evolve and move through several phases that often shift rapidly from one phase to another. It points out the effect of one small shift in the course of events on typically cascading subsequent processes. *Tipping points* refers to the critical juncture of an ongoing pattern of interactions when one seemingly slight shift results again in cascading subsequent effects that reverberate going forward in the system in focus—such as in the interactions of all those involved in a crisis. Both chaos and tipping points are key concepts to be explained more in Chapter 2.

The Cocoanut Grove fire itself started from one small match. It evolved into a vicious cycle linked with a set of factors that moved all involved with the crisis to the edge of a virtual cliff, a tipping point. As we will see, such tipping points are critical triggers for crises, as well as windows of opportunity for innovative and effective current and future interventions.

For example, there were multiple factors waiting for The Cocoanut Grove fire crisis to tip into positive results. The hospitals in Boston were unusually well prepared, having just conducted a major disaster drill with 300 mock patients preparing for a potential World War II attack by Germany on the East Coast. Penicillin had just been approved for mass use and was rushed to Boston for its first successful major implementation. The first major use of a blood bank helped save lives. The first use of emergency triage systems to direct the most effective treatment to those with the greatest potential to survive was gradually implemented and used going forward. New ways of caring for both burns and smoke inhalation were also tipped into use by the urgency of the situation. Each of these processes will be discussed presently as examples of the evolution of crises in open social systems, of chaos and catastrophe theory as they relate to crises and crisis intervention, and of what Malcolm Gladwell (2006) popularized in his best-selling book, *The Tipping Point: How Little Things Can Make a Big Difference.*

Finally, two psychiatrists were pulled in to treat survivors of the Cocoanut Grove fire: Erich Lindemann and Gerald Caplan. The work of Lindemann (1944) and Caplan (Caplan, 1961, 1963; Caplan & Caplan, 2000) initiated the systematic study and treatment of crises and their sequelae. Lindemann initiated the systematic treatment of acute grief and anticipatory grief through his treatment and study of survivors of Cocoanut Grove. His work began the study of response patterns around crisis points, complex grief, and trauma, including the classic pattern of mastery by avoidance and its treatment that we will discuss in Chapter 7. Following his involvement with the Cocoanut Grove fire, Caplan might be considered the father of crisis intervention, as he advocated for it to be included as a funded and mandated intervention in the Community Mental Health Center Act of 1963.

DEFINING CRISIS

Caplan (1961) offered a relatively straightforward definition of *individual crisis* by saying,

> People are in a state of crisis when they face an obstacle to important life goals—an obstacle that is, for a time, insurmountable by the use of customary methods of problem solving. A period of disorganization ensues, a period of upset, during which many abortive attempts at solution are made. (p. 18)

Caplan's definition fits well with the positions of this book. However, a review of a range of definitions and discussions of crisis and the goals of crisis intervention shows what we will discuss as a basic problem extending beyond simple definitions but further into the practice of crisis intervention itself.

Misguided Assumptions

Many scholars and practitioners have offered definitions of crises over the years and in different formats. James and Gilliland (2016) offered an excellent overview of many of these definitions and approaches to crisis, presenting nine different definitions and numerous perspectives on crisis and crisis intervention. What most all of them share is (a) a focus on imbalance caused by crises and (b) the need to restore that assumed balance. Some examples are terms such as psychological disequilibrium, disturbed homeostatic balance, system disequilibrium, sudden disequilibrium, and restoring persons to a state of homeostasis or equilibrium, with the goals of restoring balance and returning people and systems to previous, precrisis stable states (James & Gilliland, 2016). These basic assumptions reflect premises that, upon reflection, simply run counter to the situations we continuously encounter in the open social systems within which we all work as helping professionals. Assuming that, for instance, the precrisis relationships in battering couples, in child abusing families, or in a suicidal person's life situation are stable and that the people in these crises should be returned to that precrisis state makes little sense. Few would agree, yet these implicit goals remain unchecked and unexamined. In all of these cases, those involved need to move out of the vicious cycles of their crises and move beyond the situations that shaped and precipitated them.

While it is difficult to overestimate the cascading positive impact of Lindemann and Caplan, their influence introduced some basic flaws into how we understand and intervene in systems in crisis that persist today. Put simply, as medically trained professionals, they introduced the correct idea that crises inevitably occur in the context of systems (Caplan, 1961, 1963; Caplan &

Caplan, 2000; Lindemann, 1944). However, true to their medical training, they employed a *biological* model of systems rather than one suited for *social systems* of human interaction. Again, simply put, their biologically based view assumed that all systems were based on the principle of *homeostasis* and balance for their life. When the imbalance of a crisis occurred, the forces of homeostasis sprang into action to restore the precrisis stable state. This model of systems has classically been referred to by Walter Buckley (1967) as a structural or organismic level of systems best applied to living biological systems yet not to the sociocultural process-based systems addressed by all mental health and social service practitioners. These levels are discussed next.

System Levels

According to Buckley's (1967) analysis of system levels, there are three qualitatively different levels of systems that operate on very different principles. These levels are as follows:

- *Mechanical systems* are the most basic level of systems and consist of non-evolving elements like machines or houses of cards. These mechanical systems work on the principle of equilibrium. *Equilibrium* refers to a strict balance of a system that is intolerant to change or disturbance. Mechanical systems tolerate little input from outside the system, such that even slight differences from the strict equilibrium of the system, like touching a house of cards, can destroy the system itself. This is strict negative feedback, or a sensitive attention to maintaining a strict structure.

- *Organismic systems* are more complex, evolve, and require exchanges of things with the outside systems, such as food, water, and air to live and grow. These biological systems operate on homeostatic mechanisms to maintain the life of the system—as in body temperature, where sustained temperatures either above or below the set point for that body usually lead to death. Homeostatic balance is thus crucial to the life of the system. These biological systems are governed by more flexible negative feedback that tolerates some fluctuations, yet always reduces deviation from the set point and back to a norm.

- *Sociocultural process-based systems* are the most complex and are shaped by language and social convention. They thrive on the exchange of information to shape their interaction and they are consistently evolving. Process-based systems have positive feedback as their overriding quality. With positive feedback at their core, these systems constantly grow and evolve. These are the type of systems that are the focus of all our work as practitioners addressing crises and doing crisis intervention. These are the sociocultural systems in which we all live.

PROBLEMS WITH THE TRADITIONAL VIEWS OF CRISIS

This shift to discussing process-level systems as we move forward will require us to flesh out the qualities and relatively newer theories of open process-based systems. Chapter 2 will lay out an alternate theory like Buckley's (1967) sociocultural process-based system level. It will form the foundation of all that follows in this book and correct some basic errors causing cascading problems and missed opportunities. However, it will help to first summarize the problems of the traditional view on crisis and crisis intervention as follows:

- **Assuming stability versus change:** When we assume that all life is stable, and a crisis creates instability, then our task in crisis intervention is to return things to their prior stable state. However, all human systems are in a constant process of change, and our job in crisis intervention is to use the current perceived crisis to tip that process in new and desired directions.

- **Perceiving danger not opportunity:** When assumed stability is disrupted by a crisis, the current models implicitly draw us to see the danger of system collapse—as when a house of cards is disturbed threatening collapse, or when high fever or freezing cold threatens death to our body. All efforts are drawn into reducing the danger. However, when crises are seen as challenging transitions in the ongoing flow of life, our focus turns to facilitating new directions, previously less likely.

- **Assuming change is mainly gradual versus rapid:** Current and past views of change viewed it through a sort of Darwinian lens assuming that all change is gradual and linear across time. Current systems-based models across disciplines have shifted our understanding of change. The now-popular notion of the *butterfly effect* played out in the movie, *Jurassic Park*, in the rebirth of dinosaurs in the story, and in the classic movie, *It's a Wonderful Life*, which showed the cascading effects of seemingly small events in George Bailey's life in both positive and negative ways. These films are prime examples of how large effects can be started by seemingly small tipping points. Or the momentous fall of the Berlin Wall, which might never have been predicted, can now be traced to a confluence of apparently small shifts. Crises and rapid change are, in fact, common, and the process of change model will help practitioners expect equally rapid resolutions of each crisis as they are viewed through this same process lens.

- **Assuming reality is stable and fixed versus cocreated through process:** When we assume that we all share similar understandings of the nature of the world, we are drawn into implicit judgments of what is the norm, right, and correct. This is another byproduct of the current and traditional view of systems on which crisis intervention is based. When we embrace the idea that reality is relative to context and interactions, we begin to appreciate the need for *flexibility* and *fit* in how we approach each crisis. Practitioners are reminded to flex and adapt their own views and identities to fit the lived experiences of the people and systems with which they engage. This is a foundation of the process view and not an afterthought as in current and past approaches.

- **The importance of context:** Most current and past crisis approaches pay little attention to context in terms of language, culture, and traditions in shaping the patterns of crisis and their potential resolution. Popularly, we have awakened to the idea of diversity as it shapes our worlds. However, current texts on crisis intervention address diversity as an add-on or afterthought rather than as a foundation of how to intervene. The process of change model attends to context in all its varied elements as a foundation of how to understand each crisis and then how to intervene most appropriately to facilitate change within context.

- **The need to unify all crises within an appropriate model of change:** Current approaches to crisis and crisis intervention treat each different crisis as separate entity. Crises such as sexual assault, domestic violence, acute grief, suicidality, and trauma, for example, are explained and treated differently. There is no link among them for practitioners to use as a guide. The process of change model described in this book links all of these and others (a) by explaining the underlying patterns common in all perceived crises and (b) by supplying an overriding roadmap to intervene across them all. Although the situations and contexts will be unique to the nature of the crisis, the patterned response of all involved around the event will become predictable and will help shape positive resolutions in each case.

FOLLOWING THE PROCESS OF CHANGE

Each of the problems just described is resolved by adopting what is now called a process-based, or process of change, perspective on human interactions, problems, crises, and their resolution. However, before laying out practice guidelines for doing crisis intervention through the process of change model, we need to visit the theory and research forming the foundation of its view. Chapter 2 will lay this foundation.

2 THE THEORY BASE FOR THE PROCESS OF CHANGE MODEL IN CRISIS INTERVENTION AND BRIEF THERAPY

This chapter lays out the nature of the systemic and contextual process of change. Chapters 3 and 4 will then show how it applies to doing crisis intervention across a wide range of separate crises. Lakoff (2014) said that we have no language to describe systemic or circular change, so it is crucial that we look at the origin of the idea of process. To help with this, we will refer to several popular resources as they translate the most recent research on the process of change into more easily understandable terms. Along this journey, we will explain the basis of feedback; stability and change; how threat breeds rigidity; why creative change is often paradoxical; the importance of context and language in shaping crises; the history of a process view of the world and how it relates to chaos, catastrophe, and repeated patterns of flow in our interactions; how people are drawn into the vortex of crises through attractors; and, finally, how all of this merges into what we call the *process of change model*.

https://doi.org/10.1037/0000445-003
Crisis Intervention: Using Tipping Points to Achieve Transformative Change in Therapy, by J. S. Fraser

FEEDBACK IS THE HEART OF SYSTEMIC CAUSATION

We are all most familiar with direct, linear cause and effect. That is, A influences B, which influences C. Billiard ball A hits ball B and drives it into the pocket. Yet systemic causation is all about *feedback*. A influences B, which turns back to change A into A', which then feeds forward to influence B into B', and so on in a circular pattern.

There are two major types of feedback, positive and negative. Simply speaking, *negative feedback* reduces deviation from a given norm or set point, such as when we maintain our body temperature by sweating when hot and shivering when cold. *Positive feedback*, on the other hand, amplifies input or difference from a starting point, such as when a microphone is placed too close to a speaker system and amplifies sounds repeatedly until the characteristic screech comes out of the speaker.

However, in most systems, negative and positive feedback are integrated in many ways. For example, what might happen if the windows and doors are left open on a hot day with the air conditioner running? The air conditioning will come on to initiate negative feedback and cool the room. Yet, with the windows remaining open and letting more hot air in, the room will continue to heat up and the air conditioning will thus work all the harder to cool things down. What we will get is a *runaway* in the system: the more the cooling unit tries to cool the area, the more it fails and so on until either someone closes the windows and doors or the cooling system breaks down. Such negative and positive feedback loop interactions are an essential component of most crises. For example, with posttraumatic stress reactions, often the more we try to "remember to forget" a traumatic event, the more that effort keeps that trauma in mind, and the resulting distress triggers our repeated efforts to repress it, in the classic vicious cycle posttrauma escalating distress.

THE QUEST FOR A STABLE AND PREDICTABLE WORLD

The problems embedded in traditional approaches to crisis intervention stem from our common understanding and experiences of our world. Most of our daily routines repeat familiar patterns, such as when we go to bed, when we rise, when we eat, what we expect from our interactions with friends and family, and how safe we feel within these patterns. In essence, our language and our experiences offer us a safe and existentially comfortable view of our world. All of our ideas and experiences of the world seem to confirm this. When we experience a crisis, we thus try to settle things down to our imagined precrisis stable life, whether or not this can be said to be existentially true. John Briggs and F. David Peat (2000) suggested that

> We're all necessarily conditioned by society. Our conditioning lays out, with apparent certainty, a seemingly complete picture or map of what reality is and how we're supposed to act in it. We are trained to accept and move about in this reality from the moment we emerge from the womb. (p. 20)

Grant (2021) agreed, saying,

> [We] often prefer the ease of hanging on to old views over the difficulty of grappling with new ones. . . . Questioning ourselves makes the world more unpredictable. It requires us to admit that the facts may have changed, that what was once right may now be wrong. . . . Psychologists call this seizing and freezing. We favor the comfort of conviction over the discomfort of doubt. (p. 4)

We have also learned, through being taught Darwinian evolution, that change is always linear and takes some time. Sudden change and rapid resolutions seem to be a rare exception. This couldn't be farther from the truth.

MAKING SENSE OF OUR CHAOTIC WORLD

Fortunately, in recent years, there have been quite a few popular, *New York Times*–bestselling books we can turn to for help. These books include *Chaos: Making a New Science* by James Gleick (2008), *The Tipping Point: How Little Things Can Make a Big Difference* by Malcolm Gladwell (2006), *Think Again: The Power of Knowing What You Don't Know* by Adam Grant (2021), and *Thinking, Fast and Slow* by Daniel Kahneman (2011), among others.

- In *Chaos*, Gleick (2008) described the evolution of a new science and mathematical models to study and explain how change most often is shaped by small shifts followed by cascading patterns, and how those patterns are drawn into repeating cycles at larger and smaller scales. We will revisit this when we discuss the repeated patterns of violence in interpersonal partner violence (Chapter 8, this volume).

- In *The Tipping Point*, Gladwell (2006) made the case across a wide array of examples of how one seemingly small and innocuous trend can create a groundswell of response, similar to the infectious disease model of the spread of a pandemic. As we will see in Chapter 6, suicidal thoughts can cascade into a series of actions and reactions in the lives of those involved to eventually lock in confirmed intent to die at one's own hand.

- In *Think Again*, Grant (2021) used the escape fire example of Wag Dodge in the Mann Gulch wildfire (described in the Introduction, this volume) at the beginning of his book to explain a key idea: "Under acute stress, people typically revert to their automatic, well-learned responses" (p. 5). This is the core tenet of the explanation of crises and crisis intervention in the process of change approach to crisis. For example, early descriptions of what was termed "battered woman's syndrome" described repeated patterns of tension building, violence, attempts to placate, and respite, followed by a repeat of the same pattern with likely greater and more frequent repetitions (Walker, 2016). What is "tried-and-true" often not only doesn't solve the dilemma but also makes it worse.

- Daniel Kahneman's (2011) book, *Thinking, Fast and Slow*, resonated with Grant's (2021) perspectives in *Think Again*, as he demonstrated time and again how what we learn is typically effective as again, tried-and-true makes it seem paradoxical to choose another and often opposite alternative when under stress and threat. We will explain this more in the upcoming section on paradox, and further link it to other classic theories such as the threat rigidity hypothesis, of conservative responses under threat, and the ideas of first- and second-order change relating to the paradox of creative and effective solutions under threat and risk.

All of these books have been number one best sellers, so they certainly must have made some sense of this process of change perspective. So, let's look at how they have explained things. Maybe the most powerful and award-winning example is that of Kahneman's (2011) *Thinking, Fast and Slow*.

STABILITY AND CHANGE

Daniel Kahneman received the Nobel Prize in economics in 2002 and the 2013 Presidential Medal of Freedom for work that he and colleague Amos Tversky did on decision making under risk (Kahneman & Tversky, 2013). This type of decision making is exactly what confronts us all when we are faced with a crisis. In essence, Kahneman and Tversky put forward an explanation of how we tend to build an eventually unchallenged worldview in given domains and then stick to it in crises and under perceived risk despite facts suggesting other more successful choices. Labeling these constructs System 1 and System 2, they showed across a wide range of systems how repeated quick decisions (of System 1) slowly feed into a more general repository about similar situations (System 2). The two systems then move forward in a reciprocal self-confirming way until a unique situation arises (call it a crisis for our purposes). With the perceived requirement of quick decision making in these risky situations, typical System 1 choices are made despite the facts that those choices may not only not work but also may make situations worse. Systems 1 and 2 are constantly in operation: System 1 is continuous and System 2 is essentially in the background. System 1 continually generates suggestions for System 2 (impressions, intuitions, intentions, and feelings). If endorsed by System 2, impressions and intuitions turn into beliefs, and impulses turn into voluntary actions. Thus, under perceived threat in a crisis, we are most likely to respond in overlearned ways despite their effectiveness. However, accurate intuition is also effective in most circumstances, and that is why the ingrained beliefs and related actions and choices of System 2 persist as tried-and-true.

Once patterns are ingrained through interactions of Systems 1 and 2, they are hard to break. They take concerted System 2 effort to break by *taking perspective* and *slowing down*. The solutions are often *counterintuitive* or paradoxical from the original now-automatic assumptions. For those who have learned to drive on ice, an example of learning a paradoxical solution is overlearning the counterintuitive actions to turn into a spin and not press on the break, rather than impulsively trying to stop and turn out of the spin. Another good example discussed earlier (Introduction, this volume) is the forest service teaching smoke jumpers to set back fires to step into to save their lives. As we noted, Grant (2021) said, "Under acute stress, people typically revert to their automatic, well-learned responses" (p. 5). He pointed to the Mann Gulch wildfire as an example of how correct solutions often appear paradoxical at first.

THE THREAT RIGIDITY HYPOTHESIS

Kahneman's locked rigidity in the effects of Systems 1 and 2 echoed a set of observations and principles long applied under the term, *threat rigidity hypothesis* (Kahneman & Tversky, 2013). These observations were first put forward by Staw et al. (1981) as a thesis that has since been confirmed and used in the organizational literature and beyond for decades (cf. Chattopadhyay et al., 2001; Staw et al., 1981). This thesis suggested that "a threat to the vital interests of an entity . . . will lead to forms of rigidity" (Staw et al., 1981, p. 502). In simple terms, systems under perceived threat often initiate a vicious cycle in which increasingly conservative decisions are made under a survival focus (versus a coping focus), external information is less sought out, central decision making evolves, rigid rules are followed, and the system spirals down.[1]

---

[1]At this writing, the current analyses of Russian army defeats in their initial invasion of Ukraine have been in part attributed to rigid central command traditions as opposed to the Ukrainian army's decentralized decision-making structures offering flexible and creative choices on the front lines despite overwhelming odds.

Of course, this cycle may end if flexibility enters, and external ideas and perspectives send the cycle's trajectory toward coping in a new and more creative way. One might see this as the result of effective crisis intervention. However, such flexibility and openness are rare on their own during the crisis of perceived threat.

PARADOX AND CREATIVE CHANGE

Nearly 50 years ago, Watzlawick, Weakland, and Fisch coined the terms *first-* and *second-order change* in their classic book, *Change: Principles of Problem Formation and Problem Resolution* (Watzlawick et al., 1974). They proposed that our usual problem-solving modes typically function well within their common premises, assumptions, and rules of interaction in our daily lives. They operate in terms of first-order change principles in that continual actions within these rules and assumptions are mutually self-reinforcing and perpetuate the system going forward. When confronting more unique situations or crises, first-order solutions are quickly applied over and again until the situation is resolved. Sometimes, and truly oftentimes, this is all that is called for, and that's why these first-order patterns persist. However, at other times, a change of the premises and rules of the systems is imperative: This is what Watzlawick et al. (1974) called second-order change, or a change in how the parties deal with change. As noted earlier, this change is most often experienced as counterintuitive or paradoxical. Thus, practitioners' job is to help make these paradoxical solutions make sense to those in crisis.

Watzlawick et al. (1967) said, "Paradox may be defined as a *contradiction that follows correct deduction from consistent premises*" (p. 188, emphasis added). The idea of paradox lies in the premises or assumptions on the way things are, and not in the action itself. There is no action or instance that in and of itself is paradoxical. The idea of paradox depends on our assumptions.

Most solutions in crises, whether tried by clients or those directly involved or by practitioners, are paradoxical from the position of the original common assumptions of those facing the crisis. Making such paradoxical shifts with those in crisis will mean helping all involved make sense of such counterintuitive solutions. This will become more evident as we move to Chapters 3 and 4 on interventions and through the chapters in Part II addressing a wide range of different crises (cf. Fraser & Solovey, 2007b). Yet, what is this process view, where did it originate, and what have we learned about open systems like those we live in as they move forward and confront stress?

THE HISTORY OF A PROCESS VIEW OF OUR WORLD

In an earlier publication, I discussed the history of a process view as a different paradigm from the more deterministic linear perspective that underlies most of our traditional views of the world compared to a nonlinear process-based view of crisis, chaos, and catastrophes (Fraser, 2018). Discussing the history of a process perspective, I noted that in ancient Greece, Heraclitus launched this approach in his dictum, "everything flows." Recall his often-repeated statement that we cannot step into the same river twice—it is always flowing and changing. This is like the first-order changes and the continual interactions of Systems 1 and 2, discussed earlier in this chapter. In ancient China, Lao Tzu (ca. 500 BC) in his Taoist philosophy stated that change is constant rather than stable; sometimes change moves slowly and other times rapidly, but it is always flowing and changing in interaction within context (Hinton, 2015). His Taoist philosophy, often referred to as the *watercourse way*, aligns with Heraclitus's river metaphor generated in different places and times on the other side of the world from each other.

Moving forward, and sticking with philosophical views, the work of Alfred North Whitehead (1861–1947) in his seminal book, *Process and Reality* (Whitehead, 1978), has become synonymous with the process view in recent times. We won't linger too long with this philosophical side trip, yet this view of our world has been emphatically confirmed in the most recent research on chaos and catastrophe theories and the nature of our constantly changing worlds. As a summary of Whitehead's process view, Nicholas Rescher (1996) said about a process perspective that the "guiding idea of this approach is that natural existence consists in and is best understood in terms of *processes* rather than *things*—of modes of change rather than fixed stabilities" (p. 7, emphasis added). Rescher also suggested the following:

- Process philosophy "is really less of a theory than a point of view taking the line that one must prioritize processes over things and activities over substances. . . . Process philosophy thus prioritizes change and development in all of its aspects over fixity and persistence" (p. 35).

- Process in this view represents "a coordinated group of changes in the complexion of reality, an organized family of occurrences that are systematically linked to one another either causally or functionally. . . . Processes are correlated with occurrences or events: Processes always involve various events, and events exist only in and through processes" (p. 39).

- Processes may also evolve over time and can encompass changes without themselves changing. In this sense, "things" should always be viewed as processes. Therefore, a "thing" such as a river becomes an enduring entity while still flowing and changing.

- Rescher concluded that "Heraclitus was only half right: We indeed do not step twice into the same *waters,* but we can certainly step twice into the same *river*" (pp. 52–53, emphasis in original).

This philosophizing may appear too abstract and too far from the topic at hand as crises and crisis intervention. However, this point of view will be important to our positions on crisis and crisis intervention as we move forward to see how it has been confirmed in recent research on the nonlinear and systemic world in which we live. Far from treating crises as anomalies to be restabilized, we should instead expect seemingly unexpected changes like crises and should embrace them as the stuff of creative transformation in our lives. In fact, predictable constancy is more likely a brief interlude in the chaotic and changing world that is our life.

PROCESS AND CHAOS

The term *chaos* seems like something describing the aftermath of a terrible crash—something random and completely without order. However, the term, *chaos theory,* has come to be applied to a sophisticated mathematical approach to studying and mapping the type of things that traditional approaches had thought to be simply too random to measure. As noted earlier, Gleick (2008) first brought this to the attention of the general public in *Chaos.* Briggs and Peat (2000) explained that "the scientific term 'chaos' refers to an underlying interconnectedness that exists in apparently random events. Chaos science focuses on hidden patterns, nuance, the 'sensitivity' of things, and the 'rules' for how the unpredictable leads to the new" (p. 2). It refers to the type of systems in which we all live. Chaos theory, it turns out, matches what we mentioned in Chapter 1 as Buckley's (1967) process-level systems. These open systems are often referred to as *dynamical systems.* More recent observations and experimental findings also match the historical and philosophical views of Heraclitus, Lao Tzu, and Whitehead (1978) just mentioned. As noted at the beginning of this chapter, no language has a word for circular causality, which is the essence of these dynamical systems, so it may be helpful to turn to a classic example using Heraclitus's and Lao Tzu's river metaphors.

CHAOS AND FLOW

The study of complexity, nonlinear dynamics, and chaos in open systems has modified a wide range of perspectives on the nature of systems across many areas of study. Gleick (2008) introduced the public to chaos theory in *Chaos*. In the preface, he resonated with a process view when he said, "To some physicists, chaos is a science of *process* rather than state, of *becoming* rather than being" (p. 5, emphasis added). However, Briggs and Peat (1989) did the best translation of this often complex and technical perspective through their book, *Turbulent Mirror: An Illustrated Guide to Chaos Theory and the Science of Wholeness*. They stated, "We are used to picking out such shapes as parallel lines, circles, triangles, squares, and rectangles in nature or art . . . [when] . . . [r]egular, simple orders are in fact exceptions in nature rather than the rule" (p. 110).

The study of complexity, dynamical systems, turbulence, and chaos has arisen from studying phenomena that were never that easy to study using more static, structure-dominated, and gradualist traditions. Studying, predicting, simulating, and modeling such things as the formation of clouds and weather, the turbulence of a stream of tap water as it bursts into chaotic flow, the action of the stock market, or the fight-or-flight reactions of a dog seemed ludicrous to group together much less know how to study and predict. (This, however, is exactly our focus of study as we examine the complex interactions of clients and their problems and the complex flow of crises.)

The subject of turbulence has interested great minds and scientists from the time of Leonardo da Vinci, who drew details of turbulence and its repeated spirals and vortices. Yet all of this remained on the sidelines until the development of superfast computers that allowed visual displays and simulations of these turbulent processes. What evolved was a cascade of new concepts and discoveries. Recall Heraclitus's famous example that we can never step into the same river twice and Lao Tzu's watercourse way. Their river may serve as an example of some of the concepts of the newer perspective on process and change as adapted from Briggs and Peat (1989). Sometimes it is best to visualize systemic change when we have no words for it.

Consider Heraclitus's stream flowing through a meadow in the spring. The stream's banks channel or constrain its flow. At this point, the water in the stream flows at a relatively steady, smooth rate. The width of the banks, the incline of the stream bed, and the volume of water entering the stream also determine its rate. Occasional boulders, outcroppings, and fallen trees also shape its flow at any given time. Now, let us follow the flow of this little stream as the context changes by just one factor—that of the volume of water in the stream.

The current flow of the stream initially presents a smooth, stable, linear character—for example, always returning to the same point as it flows around a large boulder for long periods. This might reflect those smooth periods in our lives when change is orderly and predictable. We are attracted back to the same recurring patterns. (Technically, this is called a *point attractor* in chaos language.)

Now consider that spring rains begin to increase the volume of water in Heraclitus's stream. While all other constraints of the stream remain the same, the flow and speed of the water increases. At some point, the pattern of water just beyond the boulder suddenly changes. (Sudden change is common at given points in such dynamical systems, as we shall see.) From the original stable point of return as the water makes its way around the boulder, the water now forms a whirlpool or vortex that cycles the water around before it makes its way forward. (Again, as we will see, spirals and vortices are also called *vicious cycles* and *virtuous cycles*, as we discuss human interaction.) This whirlpool may stay in the same place for a long time as well, like the classic vicious cycles of John, the student with panic attacks described in the Introduction (this volume). It represents the draw of similar escalating, patterned solutions. It becomes a vortex or whirlpool. (This vortex is called a *limit cycle* in chaos terms.) In human interactions, this vortex draws all involved into the attractor of solution-generated problems representing problem-generated systems, which we will discuss further in Chapters 3 and 4. The concept of an attractor and the idea of solution-generated problems and problem-generated systems will be revisited in a following section on crisis attractors.

Eventually, as warmer days of summer creep into the surrounding mountains, snow melts and adds more water to the stream. The increased volume of water increases the speed of its flow. Now, as the water makes its way to the other side of the boulder, another sudden shift occurs. The single whirlpool of the last phase begins to spin off duplicate whirlpools that make their way further downstream from the rock and begin to resemble Leonardo's drawings of turbulence. Additionally, the choppy water undergoes much faster and more irregular changes. (Again, in chaos language, these are called *butterfly attractors*.) This chaotic process resembles the escalating cycles and patterns in East Germany leading to the sudden fall of the Berlin Wall, or the various situations with the student, John, discussed earlier (Introduction, this volume) trying to control his panic.

Finally, as the speed and volume of water in the stream continues to increase, the area behind the boulder seems to lose all of its order and the rates of flow at different points vary widely. This descent into turbulent chaos seems to have lost all order, finally termed chaos in chaos theory. However, has it?

Like da Vinci's drawings of turbulence, the whirlpools tend to break down into similar and smaller vortices, which then break apart again and duplicate themselves. Thus, there is an apparent order in this chaos that is self-similar at larger and smaller levels or scales. This self-similarity has been given the term *fractal* in the literature and has gained popular fame in beautiful computer-generated illustrations of its multiple swirls and spirals in what is termed *phase space*, or the graphic depiction of the system's movements across time and space. This idea of fractals and self-similar patterns is quite important because it suggests that patterns repeat at larger and smaller levels of systems and over time. A sample of three different quarrels is likely to generalize to a couple's classic advance–retreat cycles over time. Several examples of the student's struggle to master his panic are likely to generalize to his major pattern of mastering by avoiding and controlling over time. And, as we will learn in Chapter 8 on intimate partner violence, the classic cycles of a battering relationship reflect the same repeated cycles over time as they escalate in frequency and intensity.

Each of these observations of Heraclitus's river as it moves through increasingly more intensity reflect the same phenomena we are studying as we discuss and look to intervene in crises. However, the constraints of the riverbank, and its nature and steepness, are replaced in human interactions with our language, norms, culture, and values within the context of our lives. In a word, these represent context.

CONTEXT

From the process view, *context* refers to factors that shape reciprocal interactions in which persons (individuals and groups) coconstruct their worldviews. Interactive factors include culture, language, gender, ethnicity, race, or other socializing influences as well as resulting norms. These factors channel or constrain interaction. Interaction within these constraints gradually shapes worldviews; in return, worldviews shape interactive factors or context. Returning to Heraclitus's river, we have referred to the banks of the river, for example, as context for the water. Those riverbanks both channel the water's flow and constrain it from overflowing its banks (unless torrential rains swell the flow of the waters to create a flood—the result of the broader context of the weather).

The process view on context dovetails with Buckley's (1967) description of open social systems discussed earlier. From the process view, interactions are channeled by ideas; by constructs about the way things should be done; by explanations about the nature of experience; by understandings of what constitute appropriate gender roles; by the nature of the language used and words available in that language; by norms, metaphors, folkways, and morays within the system in question; and by what is considered a problem within a given system, and what we are typically supposed to do about it. This is why a crisis may or may not be reacted to as one by different people and groups in different contexts. As opposed to the traditional approach to crisis, a crisis is not inevitably a crisis. Context must always be considered, as we will see in our approach to crisis intervention in the next chapter.[2]

Kenneth Gergen (2022), regarding this cultural context issue, suggested that "when we are fully immersed in a given tradition or way of life, its constructions are no longer constructions. When we take our realities and values as essential and undeniable, we often trample on others' values and ways of life" (p. 28). This admonition must be taken to heart for all practitioners intervening in crises. When we assume that our definitions and understandings of the world are shared with others, we may not only invite disconnections, but we may also initiate further vicious cycles where there formerly were none.

Context also shapes our ideas of what a crisis is and what to do about it. As all involved in the crisis share similar context, language, culture, values, and traditions, they all get drawn into what we will next consider, and that is the vortex of an attractor. For example, if domestic violence is treated as a personal relationship issue, others may feel it only polite not to intervene. But when it is seen as an example of power-dominant misogyny, others are more likely to rush in to rescue. Both responses may, of course, have built-in problems, as we will eventually discuss in Chapter 8 on intimate partner violence. We will see that similar patterns recur around suicide, grief, mourning, and more. Yet, what do we mean by the term attractor?

---

[2]Years ago, when I was teaching a graduate course in crisis intervention focusing on suicide, a Japanese student reacted by saying that in some of his cultural traditions such as Hara Kiri, suicide was viewed as an honorable act. In the same class, a student from Uganda reflected that in some rural villages in her own country, a family's hut would be destroyed, and the members banished from the village if a family member had killed themselves. Cultural traditions shaped their members' views and responses to even such an assumed crisis as suicide.

CRISIS ATTRACTORS

Briggs and Peat (1989) concluded that, "We habitually see the cosmos from the point of view or order . . . [yet] . . . [w]e could imagine our familiar order as but an island of intermittency in the midst of a universe-large strange, or chaotic, attractor" (p. 63). From a chaos theory perspective, the ongoing interactions or patterns of a system are mapped onto what they term a phase space. Therefore, patterns of process can be represented as picture patterns of an ongoing flow of interactions. This is like our example of Heraclitus's and Lao Tzu's river as it flows in phases toward turbulence as the force of water in the river increases. As we saw in that river, there were rapid shifts to relatively stable vortices that drew in and shaped or attracted the flow of water around them. The constraints of the river and its flow and velocity caused these successive vortices or attractors to draw all water around into their successive patterns. Briggs and Peat (1989) defined an *attractor* in this way: "An attractor is a region of phase space which exerts a 'magnetic' appeal for a system, seemingly pulling the system toward it" (p. 36). In the constraints of our river, increased flow and velocity created a sequence of attractors from the smooth flow of a point attractor, suddenly to the limit cycle of the vortex behind the rock as flow and volume increased, to the butterfly attractor of those whirlpools breaking off and flowing randomly and colliding downstream, and, finally, to the turbulence on intense flow and volume of chaos. At each phase, the water flowing along is "attracted" or drawn into each successive whirlpool, for example, and the shift from one type of attractor is equally sudden as the force and volume reaches the next critical point.

The idea of crisis attractors will be revisited over and again in succeeding chapters. A key point is that within cultural context, the way each crisis is defined and thus responded to will create a *crisis attractor*, or a vortex into which all involved will be drawn—including clients, involved others, and practitioners. It is for this reason that understanding the language and cultural contexts for each crisis and learning the literature on that crisis in its observed context will help us both understand and intervene in those crises efficiently and effectively. The research literature on the nature of each crisis will reveal those classic patterns. Furthermore, evidence-supported crisis interventions around those crisis-attracted patterns will reveal often counterintuitive pattern reversals. As we have seen, counterintuitive solutions are common in successful crisis resolutions. This will become clearer as we move into Chapters 3 and 4 on intervention and Chapters 5 through 9 on different crises in Part II. Still, there is another important element of the process of change view that we will carry forward throughout the sections of this book. This element is the phenomenon of fractals.

FRACTALS

The discovery of fractals offers a key to linking different crises with one another and to assessing the pattern of each crisis to guide its resolution. We have observed and noted fractals several times in our previous examples, yet they are important enough to deserve their own treatment.

Merriam-Webster (n.d.-a) defined a *fractal* as follows:

> This term was coined in 1975 to describe shapes that seem to exist at both the small-scale and large-scale levels in the same natural object. Fractals can be seen in snowflakes, in which the microscopic crystals that make up a flake look much like the flake itself. They can also be seen in tree bark and in broccoli buds.

Fractals are infinitely complex patterns that are self-similar across different scales; they are never-ending and repeating. Clouds, mountains, coastlines, cauliflowers, and ferns are all natural fractals. These shapes have something in common—something intuitive, accessible, and aesthetic. The nautilus shell, meteorological patterns such as hurricanes, spiral galaxies, the spiral of pinecones, and sunflowers all include spiral fractals. Broccoli is a fine example. Every broccoli branch is identical to its parent stem. Fractal properties can also be seen in clouds.

Now, aside from being of some passing interest, most crisis patterns represent crisis attractors with nearly identical repeated patterns of human interaction as we engage in and attempt to deal with what we perceive as crises. The patterns of battering, grief, suicidal crises, and so on each represent fractal patterns as we view them through the contextual process of change. Not only do they each have their own classic patterns within their given cultural contexts, but those typical patterns repeat at larger and smaller levels of observation. Patterns of repeated attempts to resolve different crises will then repeat over time and scale. Therefore, assessing each crisis by observing at least three or more cycle patterns across time and scale will give a clear idea of the nature of the crisis patterns (or fractals) and offer clear directions for intervention.

CATASTROPHE THEORY

Next we turn to the idea of catastrophes. Like our discussion of chaos, when we think of a catastrophe, we think of an overwhelming, cataclysmic event—the crash of an airplane, the sudden eruption of a volcano, or the devastation of a sudden earthquake. Most basic definitions define *catastrophe* as an event causing great and often sudden damage or suffering. Although we will address these sorts of catastrophes in Chapter 5 on trauma, the meaning of the word we are about to turn to here within the study of nonlinear systems is somewhat different.

The changes which initiate crises are often rapid, no matter what their source. Their resolution may be equally rapid. Across the history of sciences, and certainly in the social sciences, there has been a bias toward gradualism, or the assumption that all change is slow, rational, and orderly in a Darwinian fashion (Prigogine & Stengers, 2018). In recent years, across a broad range of scientific areas, there has been a growing realization that rapid, all-or-nothing change and the emergence or pattern from chaos are much more common than once thought (Gleick, 2008; Prigogine & Stengers, 2018). The concepts of catastrophe theory in mathematics and the social sciences (Zeeman, 1976), bifurcations and rapid change in chemistry (Prigogine & Stengers, 2018), flow patterns and rapid shifts in physics (Platt, 1970), punctuated equilibrium and process in paleontology and cultural anthropology (Gould & Eldredge, 1972), and chaos theory across sciences (Briggs & Peat, 1989, 2000) all indicate that major system changes are capable of occurring in rapid, discontinuous jumps.

These phenomena are seen in such things as the flow of a stream following the slight shift of a reed or a rock; the rapid, discontinuous jumps in the development of crystals; the growth of entirely new chemical combinations rather than a return to former chemical states following the agitation of high heat; the appearance of major new evolutionary animal life forms in relatively short periods of time without expected Darwinian evolutionary links; or the decision point phenomenon for a threatened dog where only slight variations will determine whether it will attack or turn and flee. Thus, rather significant changes in system patterns are not only possible but also highly probable at crisis points.

Returning to basic definitions, *Encyclopedia Britannica* (n.d.) defined *catastrophe theory* as "a set of methods used to study and classify the ways in which a system can undergo sudden large changes in behavior as one or more of the variables that control it are changed continuously." In essence, this is what was happening in Heraclitus's river each time the flow and volume of the river reached its next critical point, and it suddenly jumped to its next state or set of cycle patterns. This is also what we saw at the fall of the Berlin Wall (described in the Introduction, this volume), when enough misinformation reached the public, and the wall guard made a choice to open the wall after becoming frustrated with his superiors. It also relates to how and why a great number of crises occur, and how practitioners may intervene to redirect crisis cycles relatively quickly into new positive directions.

Another example may be found in a movie depiction of a potential suicide. Those of us who remember the movie, *Forrest Gump* (Zemeckis, 1994), may recall Forrest's lifelong friend from childhood, Jenny. Eventually Jenny's life spun down to the point where she considered suicide by standing on a balcony railing to jump over and kill herself. Many events and poor choices gradually led to this tipping point for her where suicide seemed the only answer. This was a chaotic point in her life. Any number of slight shifts could have moved her one way or another. A gust of wind might have blown her over to her death. Someone below might have called out for her to stop, and, looking down, she may have lost balance and tumbled to her death. In the film, Jenny recalled the constant validation of her childhood friend, Forrest. With that memory, she stepped back off the balcony and back into Forrest's life. Points of extreme chaos are just like this.

Zeeman (1976) helped to popularize the concept of catastrophe theory nearly 50 years ago in his classic article, "Catastrophe Theory." He translated the pioneering work of mathematician, René Thom, and the early applications of zoologist, Konrad Lorenz, into relatively clear pictures and definitions of discontinuous, all-or-nothing change. Lorenz's classic observations of the fight-or-flight behavior in dogs offer a frequently used example. Very simply, the two emotions of rage and fear can be easily observed and measured in dogs as they encounter another dog or stranger like a mail deliverer, with mouth opened, teeth bared, and ears flattened. If no fear element emerges, the dog is more and more likely to attack and bite (much to the distress of mail deliverers over the years). However, if fear factors increase gradually (like the size of the dog approaching), the dog's behavior may tumble over a critical cliff (or cusp), resulting in immediate flight as the dog chooses to run. The key observation is that smoothly increasing changes, under the right situation, can lead to very sudden all-or-nothing change. This is simply one more key element of the open systems perspective of the contextual process of change approach at the core of the new approach to crises and crisis intervention in this book. Rapid all-or-nothing change is common, especially at the tipping points of crisis.

A small difference may make a great difference when all things may be equally probable during high turbulence. These are examples of tipping points as catastrophes. Rapid all-or-nothing change may result from one simple nudge at such tipping points. This point should also be remembered as a guiding principle for all of us doing crisis intervention. A potential, comparatively minor therapeutic intervention may very well result in a rapid shift in a positive direction out of the vortex of the crisis.

What this all means is that crises are relative to the observer. The observer's context of culture, language, norms, and so on shape the definition and form of crises. Crises tend to be grouped into patterns of vicious cycles shaped by contextually defined explanations of each crisis and how to resolve it. They occur in repeating patterns around the same defined crisis. Crises may happen suddenly, yet they often arise from gradual changes in the systems where they occur. By the same principle, they may be resolved just as quickly. And, finally, crisis intervention will thus target pattern change. It aims to move the system out of vicious cycles of escalated failed solutions and redirect those patterns to better resolutions. All of this and more will be addressed in Chapters 3 and 4 on viewing and doing crisis intervention, respectively, through the process of change.

FOLLOWING THE PROCESS

Given the twists and turns of our discussion of systems and process theories, a summary of key points might be helpful. Within relatively open, complex systems like social relationships, the following occur:

- **Observers define crises.** There are no crises out there existing separate from the concepts, focus, and interests of observers. Whitehead's (1978) process system view suggests that everything is process. The appearance of enduring substance or structures is only a product of our limited point of view or ideas on what we are observing. The universe is a set of relationships between relationships between relationships—all of which change over time. What we view as a crisis is merely an observation of events in the process of change at a given segment of time. A patient's panic attacks, a couple's struggles, or a nation's change are all products of our focus and definitions of those interactions.

- **Rules, regularities, and constraints within open systems channel their ongoing interaction patterns.** In Heraclitus's river, the constraints of the riverbank, the steepness or angle of the river bottom, and the placement of the boulder constrained and channeled the flow of water in the stream. In human social systems, norms, social conventions, concepts, and expectations reflect the constraints of a given social system. The context of our client's lives, including their culture, language, and personal histories and identities channel the flow of their lives. (The same applies to therapists.) Shifting frames and metaphors through intervention rationales may rechannel that flow. Similarly, rechanneling participants' behavior or interactions may alter their frames, metaphors, and context. This is what we will soon discuss as transformative change in process-based crisis intervention.

- **Positive and negative feedback loops are complementary.** In response to a perceived crisis, attempts at balance through negative feedback at one level may have the successive results of creating positive escalating feedback over time. The college student's attempt to calm down in the face of potential panic may have only fed back into cycles of anxiety and growing panic. His solutions became the problem.

- **Constancy/stability and change are interrelated.** As we saw in Heraclitus's river, the water in the river might change in multiple ways while the identity of the river remained the same. The banks of the river may erode more slowly while the turbulence of the stream may increase and create sudden shifts, but the identity of the stream remains constant. Constancy and change exist at different levels while both are in the process of change. Clients' attempting the same solutions with more intensity and variations on the same theme perpetuate and escalate their problem. Their solutions become the problem and perpetuate the nature of the crisis.

- **Change is constant and can be rapid.** Stability is a product of an observer's description of ongoing process at a specific time and space in the life of a system. Yet, as in the succeeding phases in Heraclitus's stream, change can also be rapid as the system amplifies in intensity over time. This applies equally to the lives of our clients and to the life of the process of crisis intervention.

- **Small changes can have cascading large results.** The overriding effects of positive feedback loops within the regularities of an open social system will tend to amplify change over time. A misinterpreted message delivered on one night in Berlin led to the cascading and dramatic opening of the Berlin Wall. Similarly, key reframes in crisis intervention or a random difference in a client's life outside of treatment may quickly lead to problem resolution for our clients.

- **Not all small changes will initiate cascading change.** Each system has certain sensitive points of information that are more likely to create reaction. The same difference may be reacted to as a potential threat to the system, or a potential opportunity, and so on. The point is that each system has parameters that will identify a difference that may make a difference. Some call these *vulnerabilities*. This is the influence of context. In our earlier examples, the college student's panic attacks were initiated by perceived situations that threatened to make him lose control. The fall of the Berlin Wall was triggered by perceived opportunity for escape by citizens feeling trapped.

- **A small sample of current patterns may reflect much larger system patterns.** As in the fractal principle of self-similar patterns occurring at successively larger scales, a smaller sample of patterned process may suffice to surmise an overriding similar process over time. From this view, just a few examples or iterations of the college student's attempts to control his panic become emblematic of variations on the same patterned and escalating cycles over time. The successive spirals of fractal images are clear examples. This aids crisis intervention assessment.

- **The goal of crisis intervention is thus shifting patterns.** Patterns are a sample of a chosen process of interaction at a given point in time and space in the ongoing system. Furthermore, patterns repeat in self-similar cycles across time and scope. This is especially true around the attractors or vicious cycles of crises. Interdicting and redirecting these vicious cycles is the goal of crisis intervention from the process view.

3 VIEWING CRISES THROUGH THE PROCESS OF CHANGE

A process view of crisis and crisis intervention offers a useful alternative to traditional and current approaches. It presents an elegantly simple model of crisis and crisis intervention as mirror images of one another, or maybe better said, two sides of the same coin. On a client's side of the coin, crises often begin with tipping points where people respond by trying the same failed solutions over and again and end up escalating the crisis rather than resolving it. On the other side of the coin, as practitioners move closer to intervening during crises, they find they have access to similar tipping points where clients are usually more open to significantly newer solutions than ever before. When practitioners adopt a process of change view, they begin to see crises as escalating vicious cycles of well-meaning solution attempts in response to a perceived threatening change. The process model thus focuses practitioners on introducing a small shift in this problematic solution pattern and then supports the client and significant others engaged with the crisis to evolve from this difference toward resolution. For example, when someone reverses their constant attempts to repress their memory of a past trauma and instead embraces and integrates it into their life going forward, they begin mastering their distress and moving through it toward growth, as we will see in Chapter 5

https://doi.org/10.1037/0000445-004
Crisis Intervention: Using Tipping Points to Achieve Transformative Change in Therapy, by J. S. Fraser

on trauma. Applying the process model, practitioners respect and build on client worldviews and strengths. By accepting the inevitability of change and collaborating with the force of the clients' drive toward resolution, practitioners can seize the opportunity a crisis offers, while reducing the potential dangers it poses. Finally, a process view holds great potential for unifying interventions across various types of crises (i.e., suicide, interpersonal partner violence, sexual assault, or grief). A process view tends to unify crisis intervention across these different forms of crisis by focusing on shifting the vicious cycles of the attempted solutions of clients, their significant others, and, frequently, other helpers. Practitioners using the process of change model begin to realize that all crisis intervention involves initiating slight shifts in solution patterns and then building on these shifts toward resolution.

Approaching crisis intervention from the process of change view involves two steps for practitioners. The first step is to adopt the idea of rapid intervention at points of first contact (whether at a defined crisis point or not) as a *first choice* for practice. The second step is to know how to do crisis intervention from this process view. This chapter focuses on the viewing of practice from a process view, and the next chapter is on the doing of crisis intervention practice from the process of change model.

CRISIS AS A WINDOW OF OPPORTUNITY FOR RAPID INTERVENTION

Gerald Caplan is one of the founders of crisis intervention (Caplan, 1963; Caplan & Caplan, 2000), as mentioned in Chapter 1 (this volume). Throughout his work, he emphasized that crises are sharply time limited, ranging from 4 to 6 weeks from inception to some form of resolution. That resolution, in his view, may ultimately be better, neutral, or worse than the precrisis state. What happens during that time will influence the outcome. However, for decades now, the average wait time for a first visit for psychotherapy has ranged from 4 to 6 weeks. The National Council of Mental Wellbeing (2022) reported that the average wait time to access behavioral health services is about 6 weeks, but wait times can stretch into months if clients are looking for a specialist in a certain area or with specific attributes. In that same report, the National Council of Mental Wellbeing offered strong data and advocacy for rapid interventions, same-day services, and crisis services as a first choice for agencies. At this writing, however, the wait time has reportedly gotten even longer. According to a survey by the American Psychological Association (APA; 2021) psychologists reported a significant increase in demand for their services since the start of the COVID-19 pandemic. And 65% said they had no openings for incoming patients at all. One might argue that clients who go to an emergency room (ER) are always seen immediately. However, follow-up referrals from ERs to outpatient care move back into that 4- to 6-week lag time. Furthermore, depending on how clients are treated in the ER, even these first contacts may be missed chances to initiate change, as will be discussed in Part II of this volume. According to Caplan, the entire field (and certainly individuals in distress) is missing a critical opportunity (Caplan, 1963; Caplan & Caplan, 2000).

When clients present with distress or are in crisis, they are typically at optimal points for influence. Their past and current problem-solving attempts are proving ineffective or making things worse, and they are seeking alternatives (albeit they may prefer *safe havens*, similar to what they have typically done and found to be safe, rather than *risky shifts*, or changing their course to do anything new and seemingly risky at a point of perceived danger). There is a longstanding literature on how to take advantage of rapid and intense interventions at these points, as we will discuss next. As practitioners embrace more rapid access and time-effective treatment, clients are likely to find shorter waiting times for contact, and practitioners are likely to be able to seize the high motivation for change with clients seen closer to crisis points. So, what do we know of the core elements of embracing rapid access at tipping points of crises with clients?

KEY ELEMENTS OF ALL EFFECTIVE RAPID INTERVENTION

Classic reviews have shown us that improvement is proportionally greater in earlier sessions and increases more slowly as sessions increase (Howard et al., 1986), with the greatest amount of change occurring within the first six to eight sessions (M. L. Smith et al., 1980). Studies suggest that 56% to 71% of the variance related to change across treatments occurs during the early sessions of therapy (Fennell & Teasdale, 1987; Howard et al., 1993). While this may be no surprise, given our emphasis on crisis and rapid intervention, effective intervention is also a product of the intervener's point of view. In short, as Budman and Gurman (2002) advocated, planned rapid intervention and time-limited practitioners tend to do the following:

> (a) value parsimony and least radical interventions; (b) see change as inevitable in a developmental perspective; (c) emphasize client strengths and resources; (d) attempt to initiate change that will continue outside and beyond the end of therapy; (e) maintain focus on the stated problem of the client and agree on resolving it; (f) respect the client's world view as important to their problem and its resolution; (g) engage with and use resources in clients' lives; and (h) plan and evaluate outcomes. (pp. 11–21)

Budman and Gurman (2002) went on to list a set of key elements common to most all practitioners applying brief therapy approaches (see also Fraser & Solovey, 2007b). These key elements converge on what many others have suggested (cf. Koss & Shiang, 1994) and include the following:

- **Maintaining clear and specific focus:** Effective practitioners share the practice of setting and maintaining clear and agreed-upon goals. This is also highly correlated with effective therapy across treatments.

- **Engaging at a high therapist activity level:** Effective practitioners tend to be active in setting session structures, setting session agendas, taking more active and collaborative roles in planning courses of action with clients, and agreeing on homework or tasks outside sessions.

- **Making explicit use of time:** Effective practitioners typically contract for set numbers of sessions in which to address agreed-upon goals. The length and timing of sessions is adjusted, including meeting for longer sessions, meeting more often, or spacing sessions to maximize effectiveness of the therapy contract.

- **Using outside factors and systems:** In addition to consistently using home-work outside of therapy sessions, most effective practitioners engage with the multiple systems in which clients are engaged. This element includes actively engaging clients' families and social networks, communicating with other social agents involved, and collaborating with other resources such as religious or other community support networks.

- **Using episodes of care:** Most effective practitioners operate on models like those of family physicians in terms of meeting with clients for a rather intensive course of brief therapy and then having the client return to their life. Clients are encouraged to return for another course of therapy as needed.

Overall, Norcross (2002) summarized elements that correlate with success across all therapies as including (a) deliberately maximizing a working alliance with clients; (b) deliberately maximizing perceived empathy; and, finally, (c) deliberately maximizing goal consensus and collaboration. Finally, pertinent to our approach to crisis intervention is the conclusion that all effective therapy boils down to two factors—flexibility and fit. *Flexibility*, as we have seen, is crucial for all parties, including therapists, involved in crises to keep them from locking in and repeating the same failed approaches over and again in keeping with the threat-rigidity hypothesis discussed earlier (Chapter 2, this volume). Flexibility for practitioners includes being able to adapt to the worldviews of clients, while staying aware of a range of proven effective approaches for the crisis at hand and being able to flexibly move among them as needed. (This, of course, requires a clear model of how to integrate effective approaches to crises, and that is the message of this book in advocating that practitioners employ the process of change model as their guide.) Regarding flexibility, the APA Presidential Task Force on Evidence-Based Practice (2006) suggested that flexibility includes such things as honoring and engaging with clients' culture, values, language, economic resources, social support, and a range of other contextual variables. Thus, practitioners are advised to *fit* the approach with their clients that best matches the client's preferred worldview, values, language, goals, and so on. Therapists also tend to do best when they have a strong allegiance to their approach, reflected in their enthusiasm and skill in the treatment and their encouragement of the client's faith and trust in both the approach and the therapist, while being willing to flexibly adopt an alternate approach that may fit better with their clients. This was a core conclusion of several prior works tracing the process view across a variety of equally effective approaches to a wide variety of problems (Fraser, 2018; Fraser & Solovey, 2007a), and it is also at the core of the process of change model of crisis intervention and brief treatment.

All of these factors will become evident in the intervention model offered next in Chapter 4. However, before moving forward, a few important factors in how to assess crises need to be covered. The first is the origin of the trigger points for crisis, and the next is a set of important concepts on the nature of crisis patterns.

KEY CRISIS CONCEPTS

There are a number of important concepts relating to crises and their patterns. These concepts include identifying the nature of trigger points and their origin; understanding the nature of how all involved are drawn into each particular crisis; and determining common and more specific crisis response patterns across crises, and how they will guide our intervention. The general literature on crises begins by addressing the nature of trigger points, so that is a good place to start.

Trigger Points

There are several classic trigger points for crisis discussed in the crisis literature. They are variously termed developmental life crises, incidental life crises, and endemic life crises. Each of these three variants essentially refers to the origin of the trigger or tipping point of origin.

- *Developmental life crises* are those that are common to the evolution of a given social system or relationship within a specific context (e.g., the development of a classic family system with transitions like marriage, child-birth, child development phases, emancipation of children, later life, old age, death of respective parents, death of a partner, and so on). A quick reflection, however, shows that such "common" developmental phases are sharply culture bound. They will be radically changed through different religious, cultural, and economic factors. They will also change with the growing incidence of single-parent families, grandparent families, unmarried couple relationships, and gay and lesbian couples who may eventually adopt, to name but a few. However, no matter what the context for the relationship, there will inevitably be transitions that will require shifting roles and status and altering relationship patterns or establishing new ones. The idea of a developmental crisis is that these transitions are inherent in the established relationship and will occur in most relationships of that sort within each given cultural context. Whether these transitions evolve into a crisis or not depends on how those involved adapt through either assimilation of or accommodation to the transition. In terms of assimilation, the transition is easily seen as no different than the typical flow and expectations of a person's life. In accommodation, those in the system simply adjust their current and future patterns to address the transition, as when those in a family system accommodate for a child moving into adolescence or when a grandparent moves into the nuclear family later in their life for health reasons or earlier to help with childrearing. However, successive failures of these efforts typically lead to crises and familiar vicious cycles.

- **Incidental life crises**, on the other hand, represent unexpected trigger points. They are chance incidents. Events such as a mugging, sexual assault, vehicle crash, tornado, earthquake, and the like may never occur in the life of some individuals and social relationships, yet they occur seemingly regularly in others. Some of these events are shared, such as the multiple challenges of the recent COVID-19 global pandemic, tornado devastation, or, at this writing, an earthquake in the Middle East that claimed more than 50,000 lives and resulted in untold injuries and social and economic damages. Other events may seem individual, yet they are always embedded in a social context and set of relationships within which they resonate and reverberate. Sexual assault is an example in which an individual attack may have occurred, yet the sequelae may involve police, medical personnel, family, partners, friends, and more. We will introduce potential suicide as another incidental crisis (Chapter 6). Once again, whether these incidental trigger points evolve into a crisis depends on how all involved relate to it through action to assimilate or accommodate as in the developmental crisis just described. Similarly, repeated failed attempts typically result in the now classic vicious cycles of crisis.

- *Endemic life crises* are those that occur as part of repeated cycles that happen within set relationships and tend to evolve in frequency and intensity over time (cf. Fraser, 1988, 1989). They tend to be a product of the cultural context that shapes and perpetuates them. These refer to the escalating patterns of violence in a domestically violent relationship that typically increase in intensity and frequency over time. They also often occur in child sexual abuse typified by the concept of grooming, in which a perpetrator, such as an adult in some position of authority (e.g., a family member, church leader, or social group leader) uses their relationship to gradually introduce sexual talk, touching, and so on. Sexual assault and intimate partner violence are endemic crises in that they have been strongly related to what is termed as the *patriarchy* in each culture and the influence of power and control, as we will examine in Part II as we discuss these related crises. Each of these endemic relationships involves common elements that exclude outside input and close the relationship to others. Classic crisis points often occur upon discovery or disclosure. Once again, whether these patterns eventually escalate into a more intense crisis depends on the nature of the context and the responses of those directly and indirectly involved. There will be much more about these endemic crises in Chapters 8 and 9 on intimate partner violence and sexual assault, respectively.

Although the history and context for each crisis is relevant in many ways, the overall pattern of each evolving crisis remains the same. A brief reflection on the principles of open systems (cf. Fraser, 2018, pp. 70–73) affirms that in open social systems, one can get to the same end point from a wide variety of starting points (*multifinality*), and the same end may be reached from widely different beginning points (*equifinality*). As such, not all of the same developmental transitions, incidental changes, or endemically shaped interactions will result in a crisis spiral. What this means is that it is the *intervening process* that influences the course of a system. It is the pattern of repeated failed solutions that breed crises. A sample of several solution attempts in context will offer the best idea of the pattern of the particular crisis and how it might be redirected or interdicted.

Crisis Attractors

Goerner (1995) suggested an evolving ecological view of order within social systems where order grows. According to Goerner,

> [To] get new order you need three things: constraints, fluctuation, and energy. No fluctuations, no seeds for the next round of growth. No constraints, no boundary to channel growth—you never get more than random collisions. No energy, no drive, no nothing. (p. 30)

This is at the heart of a process view. For example, all people live in cultures where there are prescribed ways of expecting a loss and responding to it when it occurs. When a person feels particularly surprised and distressed by a specific event like an unexpected death or loss, they typically have a culturally prescribed way of responding to it and they need to have some sense of urgency to resolve the loss. If the loss is not felt as significant, there will be little drive for resolution. However, repeated ineffective attempts at resolution by the person, others in their life, or both will likely yield cascading patterns of ineffective resolution, including such things as social withdrawal, continual crying, and so on.

Again, crises evolve from perceived fluctuations within a domain of constraints and are fueled by the energy or force to resolve them. Both the pattern and the shape of the subsequent interactions tend to produce characteristic patterns around each type of crisis. This ordered pattern, this spiral, grows from apparently random turbulence around a perceived change. Crises, therefore, are *evolving spirals*.

In all crises, there is a perceived shift or change in what is viewed to be a safe and stable pattern. In a crisis, there are (a) descriptions and ideas of those involved with the shift, which then constrain and guide the way the shift is acted upon; (b) some significance is placed on this change wherein it may be perceived as potentially threatening and which calls for action upon it; (c) explicit and implicit goals are implied in resolving the change as described; and (d) the related sets of actions traditionally connected to the defined change are then engaged to resolve it.

As we will see in Chapter 7 on grief and loss, different cultural traditions shape our expectations around death and loss and how and when to appropriately respond to it. We will discuss in that chapter how even the death of a baby or young child, which most would find tragic, can be treated in some cultures as a blessing. However, once these elements are moved into action in attempts to recapture perceived stable safety, either the resolution or the evolution of a crisis spiral begins.

These patterns have been conceptualized as solution-generated problems, problem-generated systems, and problem patterns, both generic and specific (cf. Fraser, 1986, 1988, 1989, 2018, 2020; Fraser & Solovey, 2007b). Each is discussed next.

Solution-Generated Problems

The term *solution-generated problem* has been used several times thus far to describe the characteristic vicious cycle that often emerges when people try to negotiate change. It is a simple shorthand term for the common crisis spirals of repeated first-order changes applied within agreed-upon first-order realities. These processes are the product of the well-meaning attempts of all parties involved around a crisis point to bring it to resolution; however, these same solutions are the very elements that are contributing to its escalation.

Describing crises as solution-generated problems emphasizes that it is the solutions that are the problem; therefore, these solution patterns should be the target of change in intervention. At another level, many traditional approaches to crisis intervention may feed into these same solution-generated problems to the extent that they match the positions of the clients involved in the crisis. For example, offering all the reasons for a suicidal client to live may further distance them from a practitioner if that simply repeats what helpful others have done to no avail. Thus, for a practitioner, altering one's concepts of crisis and crisis intervention and changing therapeutic solutions may be equally important targets for change.

Problem-Generated Systems

As mentioned previously, a process view holds that there is no such thing as an invariant system that exists on its own without an observer to name it and describe it. Therefore, systems around crises may vary depending on those who become involved. The problem-generated system is a useful idea when intervening in crises. This idea can practically include and exclude those people with whom an intervenor may want to engage. A *problem-generated system* is simply composed of all of those people who are actively engaged in defining a situation as a problem and are attempting to do something about it (Goolishian & Winderman, 1988).

The problem-generated system, for instance, may include one, two, or all members of a nuclear family, depending on the situation. Such a system may emerge uniquely around a specific crisis, then dissolve at its resolution, never to interact again. In addition, such a system might involve nonfamily members such as a truant child, a truancy officer, a teacher, and a parent; or it may include a rape survivor, a nurse, an ER physician, a police officer, and a court referee. Professional helpers must always remember that when they are involved as intervenors, problem-generated systems always include themselves and their ideas about the problem and their attempts to resolve it. Problem-generated systems are the players who are involved in the solution-generated problems who all agree that the situation is a crisis and are actively engaged in attempts to resolve it.

Problem Patterns

There are two key concepts critical to understanding crises and doing crisis intervention from the process perspective. The first has been termed generic crisis patterns, and the second is specific crisis factors or patterns.

Generic Response Patterns

In following this discussion of vicious cycles and unique frames of differing realities, one might begin to assume that each new crisis pattern is likely to be unique to those individuals involved in it. To some extent this is true. There will always be more or less novel spins in each new case. However, if intervenors assume that each new crisis springs anew from nothing and is completely different than anything they had ever seen before, there would be little sense in attempting to understand or prepare for them. From a process point of view, there is a basis for expecting to find general similarities in the pattern of responses around similar types of perceived events within similar contexts. To the extent that people involved in different instances of similar events share similar ideas, language, and traditions of describing and responding to these types of difficulties, the pattern of their responses around the emerging crisis will be similar as well; this becomes a *generic response pattern.*

Generic response patterns within a given culture will generally be similar within similarly defined crises such as intimate partner violence or sexual assault and yet relatively different between cultures. The shared concepts, language, and traditions of response tend to define a set of parameters within which all who share them are drawn into a similar pattern of interaction. These patterns also serve as cautions as to how intervenors might be drawn to respond themselves if they share the same unexamined definitions, values, and traditions as their clients and thus may be drawn into the same generic patterns. When used wisely, however, the idea of generic response patterns can offer guidance on the nature of different crises, define probable goals, and describe consequent interventions that are most likely to be effective. A generic response pattern to a specifically defined crisis such as suicide or grief presents a general category of solution-generated problem patterns for each defined crisis. Generic response patterns offer the intervenor a shorthand template of what they might expect from all involved in a specific type of crisis. Therefore, it is always important for practitioners to become aware of the patterns around particular crises through research within the culture in which they are working.

Specific Response Patterns

The idea of specific response patterns serves as a balance to the templates of the generic patterns. *Specific response patterns* refer to those unique elements of each individual, family, subculture, or other context that exerts their own specific influence on how those involved define and respond to a given change. These elements may include unique aspects of ethnicity, race, gender, sexual orientation, disability, power, and other areas of diversity and their interaction, which may come into play among the people involved. These dynamics may also include the unique patterns of interaction that may have evolved between a specific couple, within a particular family, between agencies or professionals, or within a community, among other things. The nature of specific response patterns is always influenced as well by the unique characteristics of the intervenor.

In short, specific response patterns may combine with a generic pattern to give it a slightly different spin. They may, on the other hand, exert such influence as to completely override or alter an expected pattern and produce a pattern different from what is generically seen for that type of crisis. As mentioned earlier, each crisis does not spring forth uniquely from all others before it. Generic patterns around defined types of crises within given cultures do tend to exist. Therefore, it is important for practitioners to consult the literature on each general crisis with which they are involved. (This is the objective of the chapters in Part II of this book.) Yet the specific patterns of each new system must be considered because they will add the unique elements particular to each case. All of these key concepts will help to guide our discussion in Chapter 4 of how to do crisis intervention from a process of change view.

FOLLOWING THE PROCESS

How practitioners view crises will shape how they will intervene in those crises. Interventions at tipping points when clients engage with practitioners hold the elements of rapid and transformative change as they are shaped by this set of process-based ideas. The key components of viewing crises through a process lens can best be summarized as follows:

- How crises are triggered and evolve from tipping points in the lives of clients, and how they may be rapidly and effectively interdicted and turned in positive directions at the tipping points of contact with practitioners, are mirror images, or two sides of the same coin within a process view of change.

- As practitioners view crises as escalating vicious cycles, their interventions turn to understanding what is shaping the direction of those cycles, aligning with the values and goals of all involved, and introducing often small yet significant shifts in those cycles to initiate tipping points toward more positive directions and outcomes.

- As practitioners adopt a process-based view of crises, they will find that it applies in the same ways across most all variations of crises. It will serve as a unifying guide to interventions across crises as opposed to the current patchwork of approaches.

- As practitioners adopt a process-based approach to rapid intervention and brief, effective therapy, they will begin to shift their practice toward engaging with clients around their experienced crises as a first choice in practice.

- Practitioners adopting this process-based view of change will begin embracing crises as valuable windows of opportunity and as tipping points for rapid and efficient change with their clients.

- Key elements of all effective rapid intervention by practitioners include the following:
  - maintaining clear and specific focus on the presenting crisis;
  - maintaining high activity levels throughout the interventions;
  - attending to the explicit use of time in the timing of sessions, their length, and frequency of future contacts;
  - actively engaging with outside systems and resources and prescribing homework activities for all involved to initiate new pattern shifts; and
  - adopting an *episodes of care model* in which rapid and intense interventions are interspersed with periods where clients reengage with their lives.

- Tipping points that present potential triggers for crises are generally divided into developmental life crises, incidental life crises, and endemic life crises.

- Practitioners view crises as attractors for all involved, which draw everyone into similar responses and solutions that take on the characteristics of generic and classically recognized patterns within given cultural contexts.

- Practitioners look for repeated patterns within each identified crisis to determine the nature of the crisis and whether it conforms to the classic patterns of that type of crisis.

- Practitioners remain acutely attuned to the language, culture, traditions, and related aspects within clients' lives and that of the systems with which they are engaged to shape and guide their understanding of how the crisis has evolved and is maintained. They also use this understanding to align with the values and goals of all involved and to develop frames and related rationales within which to fit their interventions.

- Practitioners view all crises as a product of a perceived shift or change in what is viewed to be a safe and stable pattern. Thus, they view crises as a product of the following:
  - the descriptions and ideas of those involved with the shift, which then constrain and guide the way the shift is acted upon;
  - the significance placed on this change wherein it may be perceived as potentially threatening and which calls for action upon it;
  - the explicit and implicit goals implied in resolving the change as described; and
  - the related sets of actions traditionally connected to the defined change that are then engaged to resolve it.

- Practitioners look for two related pattens around the vicious cycles of each crisis, including the following:
  - Solution-generated problem patterns are the classic, self-perpetuating, and rigidly exacerbating solution patterns that define each crisis. Practitioners thus focus on these patterns as the main focus of intervention.
  - Problem-generated systems are the network of all parties and agents involved with each crisis who are defining the situation as in urgent need of attention and are actively engaged in resolving it (practitioners target engaging with all of those involved in these problem-generated systems as their clients).

- In each different crisis, practitioners look for two variations of potential vicious cycle patterns to identify the nature of the crisis and to guide their eventual interventions. These two potential crisis patterns break down into the following:
  - Generic response patterns are the classic and expected patterns around a given crisis within a given cultural context as described by the history of the literature that has described what might be expected in each different crisis. Practitioners may then use these expected, common response patterns and frames associated with them to guide their initial plans for intervention.
  - Specific response patterns are a product of those unique elements of the context of the crisis and the history, language, and culture of all

those involved that then tend to alter the shape and pattern of what might have been viewed as a generic crisis pattern. Practitioners remain acutely aware of these specific factors to then shape their intervention to fit those involved rather than routinely applying interventions found to fit with most generic response cycles around each given crisis.

- Finally, all of these elements of the process view of crises and crisis intervention combine to shape how practitioners view each new crisis and, consequently, how they will engage in doing crisis intervention and brief therapy according to the process of change model, which is the focus of the next chapter.

4 DOING CRISIS INTERVENTION FROM THE PROCESS VIEW

Let's turn now to how to do crisis intervention from the process view. We will start with a few cases.[1]

John came into the crisis center after having been on the phone most of the night with crisis workers who encouraged him to come in. He was suicidal. He lost his job as a security guard a few months earlier. He weighed filing for bankruptcy but felt he didn't want to stiff his creditors. Then, after a whirlwind courtship and marriage, his new wife left him. While driving, John considered slamming his car into a wall. A day earlier, he sat on his bed drinking, with his handgun from his past job as a security guard in his lap. He continued to call his bride, but she told him to back off, she needed space, and he needed to quit his crying. His family's response to his wife leaving was to say, "Good riddance," and remind him there was a lot to live for. Yet, all John wanted was to get his wife back. At the crisis center, John's therapist agreed with him that there were many reasons to die, given his situation, and argued there was time to plan that out better if he really

---

[1]All case examples are based on real clients, whose identities have been disguised to maintain confidentiality.

https://doi.org/10.1037/0000445-005
Crisis Intervention: Using Tipping Points to Achieve Transformative Change in Therapy, by J. S. Fraser

wanted to. The therapist noted that John seemed to show care for others; he had chosen not to declare bankruptcy out of concern for how it would impact his family. He also agreed that he was not an impulsive person. And if John wanted his wife back, then he would need to stay alive. As far as a plan, the therapist suggested that it might be best right now for John to give his gun to his family while both of them strategized on how to affirm his wife's request for space from him. John agreed. He went to stay with his cousin locally and stopped calling his wife. When she called, he said he was honoring her request for space. They eventually came in as a couple to sort out their relationship.

Linda and Chuck, a married couple, presented for therapy due to domestic violence issues. Chuck had called a few days earlier saying he needed to find out why he was getting so violent with his wife. The therapist saw Chuck alone first, in that he was the requesting client, then Linda alone. There had been an escalating cycle of domestic violence over the past year, increasing in severity and frequency, along with growing isolation of the couple, especially Linda, from others. Chuck told of a history of being robbed and hit over the head, using medication for a bad back, and having a habit of drinking beer and other alcohol. He wondered if those were the reasons for his violence. Linda came in with two black eyes, and she was holding her painful ribs after a violent argument days earlier. She told Chuck to get help or she might need to leave him, and that was why they were here. She also loved Chuck and simply wanted to help him. She thought he had broken her arm earlier but was too embarrassed to seek medical help. Others told her to leave Chuck, but she wanted to have someone help her to stay if she could. The therapist told her of the classic cycles of violence that may result in more serious injuries or even death. However, if Linda really wanted to help Chuck, she would agree to go down to the first floor of the hospital and have Chuck with her in the emergency room (ER) to get treatment and have him see what he had done. Chuck agreed to further diagnostic assessment for his head injury and to revise his medications. We contacted the ER staff, we told them of the couple's situation, and the couple agreed to go right down to the ER. They temporarily separated while awaiting the results of Chuck's assessments. Linda eventually left Chuck. Chuck learned his violence was caused by nothing but himself and his violent attempts to control others.

Ann came in following a sexual assault by a man she met through an online dating service. She had a history of being sexually molested by her older brother when they were younger. She told her mother about the abuse, but her mother did not believe her; she told Ann that if it had happened, then it was usually the female's fault for not watching herself. Recently, Ann had begun hearing accusing male voices telling her she was trash, and she was staying up all night arguing with them. She was afraid to tell her mother and friends of the assault for fear they would blame her, as she did herself for not being more careful. The therapist told her she was amazed at Ann's bravery in coming in and sharing all of this and commended her for her resilience now and in the past, as she survived past assaults as well as this one. Of course, this and the other assaults were not Ann's fault, but were the responsibility of the men who assaulted her. Her therapist said it was likely no mistake that the accusatory voices she heard were males, as that was the patriarchal society's message to all women. Her therapist asked her to stop arguing with the voices because the arguments were simply reaffirming them and further drawing her in. Ann and her therapist then worked out a plan for her to resume working for a local library to get out more and be less isolated. She also got a dog and began volunteering at the local animal shelter. Ann eventually confronted her mother for not believing and supporting her now and in the past. The voices subsided as she moved forward.

The day after Christmas in 2004, a massive tsunami hit Sri Lanka and the surrounding South Pacific area, killing over a quarter million people. The Western world responded by sending hordes of mental health disaster workers and therapists to help the population with their posttraumatic stress disorder (PTSD) and recovery. They trained fleets of indigenous residents and Buddhist priests in the latest Western research on the patterns of PTSD and how to respond. Individual trauma counseling was recommended. However, few intervenors had any understanding of the culture they were entering or the country's local languages, religious beliefs, and burial rituals along with the population's long history of civil war. When the local populations did not react the way the Western intervenors expected, they were confused and felt the population was "clearly in denial" (Watters, 2011, p. 75). However, Sri Lankans had become remarkably resilient, given their collectivist culture and experience surviving poverty, hardship, and war and their reliance on their religious healing traditions. The Hindu and Buddhist traditions of accepting pain as part of life and beliefs in rebirth helped most survivors accept and respect their fate and move forward together. They relied on strong family and community bonds. Taking time from their duties and important social roles for individual counseling with strangers became problematic within this collectivist culture. In essence, the Western ideas and interventions exacerbated the conditions they were supposedly trying to cure.

The first three cases are all examples of engaging with crises through the process of change. The *process of change* is a model for understanding crises in their context, engaging with all involved using their values, culture, and language, honoring their goals, and shifting vicious cycles to move them all forward. This is particularly different than most current mainstream approaches. The only exception is the last case, in which the intervenors in Sri Lanka overlooked all these elements in favor of their own views and evidence-supported models within their own Western culture and thus exacerbated problems rather than solving them.

Taking each example in turn, we can see the basic elements of the process of change view. For a start, there is always a context and history within which each crisis occurs:

- In John's suicidal crisis, he had several recent losses, and he had pinned his hopes on his new marriage.

- In Linda's relationship with Chuck, there had been a history of Chuck's power and control and his gradual isolation of Linda from others.

- For Ann, her history of sexual abuse by her brother, denied and blamed on her by her mother (and often by society), set the stage for her reaction to her recent assault.

- Sri Lanka's impoverished state, history of civil wars, collectivist culture, and Buddhist and Hindu religious views set the stage for its population's response to the disaster of the tsunami.

All crises begin with a kick point, trigger, or perceived significant shift or difference that is viewed as dangerous and likely to threaten those involved. In the cases just described, these triggers were as follows:

- For John, the trigger was his bride's second thoughts about their impulsive decision to marry.

- For Linda, it was the severe beating Chuck gave her after an argument about her going out to find him after being afraid of being left alone.

- For Ann, it was having her trust and safety violated once again as she was overwhelmed and sexually assaulted at the end of a first date.

- For the survivors in Sri Lanka, it was the unexpected death and destruction following a historic tsunami.

There is always a reaction targeting resolution of the perceived crisis by all those involved and shaped by their common life patterns, context, and history:

- For John, his immediate response was to tell his bride every day how much he loved her and how tragic it would be to lose her, trying to bring her closer to him.

- For Linda, she had always forgiven Chuck, accepted his apologies and explanations for his violent temper, then the cycle repeated. (Yet this time she did something different by demanding he seek help.)

- For Ann, her response revolved around cycles of self-blame, isolation, and then disputes with the degrading male voices in her mind.

- For the Sri Lankan survivors, their common responses were to rejoin with their families and communities, accept the distress as part of life's inevitable pain, and soften the impact of death and loss by claiming the dead were simply on a trip elsewhere.

There is an inevitable response to the solution attempts, sometimes resulting in resolution or assimilation of the perceived crisis event, yet often evolving into ongoing vicious cycles. Sometimes these vicious cycles resemble common generic patterns around the crisis according to the literature on the problem.

- In John's case, his wife reacted by feeling smothered and misunderstood, and she pushed John away more, resulting in John's classic vicious cycle of his advance to her retreat—and so the cycle evolved—resulting in John's desperation and thoughts of suicide. (This is a common advance–retreat generic pattern in many couples.)

- Linda was drawn in as a part of a classic battering cycle including the patterns of assault, loving respite and honeymoon, then growing tension, increased isolation, and, finally, another violent assault. (Recall that these cycles are fractal patterns that repeat in similar form and variation as we discussed in terms of chaos theory in Chapter 2.)

- Ann's reaction to her rape followed a common vicious cycle pattern of self-blame, within the cultural context of blaming the victim, her mother's history of blaming her, and Ann's subsequent withdrawal into herself and her disputes with the accusing male voices in her mind. (This likely reflects her draw into a patriarchal cultural context.)

- The dominant Western culture's response to the Sri Lankan people after the tsunami was to impose their own Western-based, research-supported views of how people respond to trauma and how healing and treatment is best achieved. When this did not fit with the people's response, the intervenors blamed the people for rejecting their help and redoubled their efforts to offer the same help in an escalating vicious cycle.

There are always goals for resolving each crisis by all involved. In our case examples, these goals were as follows:

- For John, it was to reestablish his relationship and regain his wife.
- For Linda, it was to help Chuck with his violence and regain safety in her marriage.
- For Ann, it was to end the persecuting voices, regain her self-respect, and feel safe again to engage with others.
- For the Sri Lankan people, it was to appropriately mourn their losses and regain their lives and routines within their families and villages.

The network of significant others involved around the perceived crisis always needs to be identified, and their positions and responses to the crisis should be considered because they contribute to the vicious cycles of the crisis or they may aid in its resolution.

- John's network was clearly his bride, yet also his family members who had engaged with him the night before over the phone. The question became how accessible and engageable each might be.

- Linda's network clearly included Chuck and his frame that his violence was a result of external causes. Yet, it also would include Linda's friends and family and, eventually, ER nurses and physicians.

- Ann's involved others appeared to be her mother and brother, yet they appeared inaccessible.

- For the people of Sri Lanka, the most accessible network around the current crisis response was that of the Western intervention teams. Beyond that, likely networks would be family, community resources, and religious figures.

Interventions inevitably target pattern shifts and reversals in the escalating vicious cycles.

- For John, it was to reverse his advance–retreat cycle with his wife, interrupt his suicidal thinking, remove danger, and reverse his patterns of isolation.

- For Linda, it was to break the battering cycle, increase safety, and reengage with her social network.

- For Ann, it was to stop and redirect her arguments with the persecuting voices, reframe herself as a strong survivor of external attacks and blame, and reverse her social withdrawal.

- For Sri Lanka's intervenors, it was to reverse their efforts to train for PTSD responses and related interventions and turn them toward accepting and respecting the natural healing traditions of the culture and religions of the country.

There is always a need to accept, respect, and utilize the views, values, strengths, and resources of those involved around the perceived crisis.

- John's value was to do right by others, to show love and respect for his wife, and to be a steady person.

- Linda's wish was for her therapist to understand her love for Chuck and to invest in helping him to stop his violence.

- Ann viewed the male voices she was hearing as essentially real and harassing so she wanted to know how to defeat them.

- The people of Sri Lanka simply wanted to have their traditions and culture respected.

Successful interventions always affirm the distress and embrace the goals and values of all involved as they turn the patterns around the crises to interdict and redirect vicious cycles. When evidence-supported interventions are used, they are always adapted and fit the parties involved.

- The pattern of others rejecting John's distress and suicidal ideation was reversed by confirming his despondence yet allowing that suicide could always be a possibility down the road if nothing worked out in his plan with the therapist. John's suicidal ideation decreased as he and his therapist collaborated on a plan to regain his wife's affection by not calling her and being less available while at his cousin's house. The family was also contacted to have them affirm John's distress and value for his marriage and keep his guns while something could be worked out.

- Linda's pattern of not seeking help and isolating was reversed by having her go to the ER for her injuries, encouraging her to do so in service of helping Chuck see the results of his violence. Chuck's wish to find out why he was violent was supported through assessments that ended up eliminating all external causes and turning to his own responsibility and need for self-management.

- Ann's vicious cycles of disputing the voices' persecution was turned by framing her engagement with them as simply giving them what they wanted. Accepting their presence as her lived experience, yet not taking the bait by arguing, opened opportunities for her to reaffirm herself and reengage socially.

- While there was no opportunity for an external source to turn the Western intervenors from their crusades to help the people of Sri Lanka, eventually their experience and some input from other sources ended their efforts.

Once a small pattern shift begins, then it is supported, amplified, and generalized and the success is attributed to those involved rather than the practitioner.

- John was congratulated for respecting his wife's need for distance, and the couple was supported in sorting out their new relationship.

- Linda was supported in her willingness to help Chuck by seeking help for herself and eventually linking with a women's group.

- Ann was commended for her strength through surviving assaults and respecting her own strength as she reengaged socially and confronted her mother.

- Western practitioners ultimately learned to honor the culture and traditions of those being helped.

All of these elements are then embedded in a more practical intervention session model to help guide practitioners through their initial contacts—the *process of change model*. We discuss this model next.

THE PROCESS OF CHANGE INTERVENTION PROCESS

The process of change model has a six-phase process that relates to the very simple ABC model (cf. Cavaiola & Colford, 2017; Kanel, 2019), with A standing for achieving contact, B for boiling things down to specifics, and C for coping actively with the crisis (Figure 4.1; cf. Fraser, 2020). The circular arrows between each phase indicate the flexibility of the model, as practitioners and clients may need to recycle to be sure they mutually understand each other and that their relationship is maintained and moving forward.

FIGURE 4.1. The Six-Step Process of Change Model

"ABC" Structure:		Six Phase Process:
(A) **Achieve Contact** With the Person or Parties	→	(1) **Relationship Establishment** ↻
(B) **Boil Problem** Down to Specifics	→	(2) **Information Gathering** ↻
	↘	(3) **Consensual Problem Formulation** ↻
		(4) **Break/Recess** ↻
(C) **Cope Actively** With the Problem As Agreed Upon	→	(5) **Problem Solving** ↻
	↘	(6) **Summary**

Refined Elements of the Six-Step Process of Change Model

In a more contemporary and systematic description of the overall process of change model, the six steps of the process of change model may be fleshed out as follows.

Step 1: Relationship Establishment

- What is the crisis? Is it acute trauma, acute grief, suicidal ideation, sexual assault, domestic violence, or another crisis? How might this crisis affect the relationship with intervenors?

- What is the context of the crisis? What are the country and culture, languages, traditions, and religious beliefs? Do they match that of the practitioner?

- What individual factors of the identified persons may create unique or specific crisis response variations? What are peoples' unique roles or status, gender differences, relationship differences, personal histories, and so on? How do these potentially modify generically expected crisis response patterns for this type of crisis?

- How does the nature of the crisis and its context, along with those involved, match with the identity, training, skills, and values of the practitioner? To what extent does the practitioner match with the nature and needs of the identified system? What needs to be changed to fit with those involved to join with them to facilitate change?

- How can the practitioner be sure to flex and fit with the client as the relationship moves forward? Therapists need to be flexible enough to adapt to the client's worldview, language, and culture and then fit their rationales and frames for intervention to make sense to the client.

Step 2: Information Gathering

- What are the strengths and resources of those involved in the crisis? How can the strengths of all involved be identified and martialed in service of change? Is change already beginning and how may this be built on?

- What are the current response patterns around this crisis, and are they escalating the problem? How are all involved reacting to the situation, what are they doing to try to resolve things, and how is this either working or making the situation worse?

- What is the literature on generic response patterns around that crisis? What are the common phases, common challenges, typical risk factors, common crisis-generated solutions, typical system reactions, and so on, and how do they apply to this case? Do they need to change, given the unique elements of those involved and their context?

Step 3: Consensual Problem Formation and Goal Setting

- Given the current response patterns around the crisis, what needs to change? What patterns need to be interrupted, shifted, reversed, reframed, and used to shift the crisis patterns in the direction of resolution? How can these fit with the current values and motivations of those involved?

- What common crisis-generated systems are involved? What does the literature and common practice inform us about helping others who may be involved in a given crisis? What do we know of their typical response patterns?

- Who in the crisis-generated system needs to be involved as a target for intervention, and what needs to be shifted in their responses? These others may include family, community, friends, school, medical personnel, or police. Shifting the response of significant others may be as important to resolution as intervention with an identified person in crisis.

- How does the potential needed intervention fit with what has been supported in the literature as effective, and how might it need to be altered to fit? Always be informed about what has been found to work with this crisis, then match it with the system and alter if needed to fit.

- Do those involved agree to the goals of the intervention? Is it stated in their own language, according to their own values and goals, and aligned with their own personal motivations to change?

- Is there agreement to move forward with a plan? Are all involved in the session on the same page with the rationale for explaining the crisis and the plan for moving forward with a new direction?

Step 4: Break/Recess
- If possible, break at least briefly to give all involved time to gain perspective. Even if the session is held on the phone or in situations where all parties must stay with one another, at least slow everyone down to gain perspective on the problem as defined to generate perspective and creative problem-solving options. If possible, discuss with a colleague before reconvening.

- Why take a break? The break serves to allow all involved to once more step out of the system to see the larger picture rather than just the smaller details.

- What should the practitioner do when all involved reconvene? Always check to see what those involved have come up with or might suggest before moving forward, and always incorporate their input into the problem-solving step to follow.

Step 5: Problem Solving and Interventions
- Engage the intervention with all involved. After assessing the patterns, goals, and needs for change, try out matching interventions and adapt and alter them with feedback from those involved.

- Reinforce and support shifts in patterns as change begins. Build on success and ascribe change to the strengths and values of all involved.

- Engage all involved along with helpful resources to support the change moving forward. Be sure to enlist supporting resources in the helping network and community to reinforce the changes going forward as the practitioners step away.

Step 6: Summary and Closure
- Prescribe "fire drills" to anticipate and create resilience against future similar challenges. Create relapse prevention strengths to harden the system and prepare for future occurrences around similar challenges.

- *Step out yet invite future contact as needed.* Frame the practitioner as a resource to be used to bolster the system's strengths and needs in the face of future challenges. Use a family physician frame, for example, to normalize the use of help as needed.

The real creativity in applying these phases comes in as the pattern shifting intervention evolves. In most cases, this pattern shift is a complete reversal of the vicious cycles around the crisis. This shift is commonly experienced as counterintuitive or paradoxical by those engaged in the crisis. It is therefore crucial for the change strategy to make sense to all involved. Thus, engaging with the language, culture, values, and invested goals and motivations of the clients and using them to frame and make sense of the counterintuitive is most important. Even when evidence-supported interventions fit best, these interventions most frequently involve pattern shifts and reversals in themselves that may seem different and even risky. Once more, the plans and strategies always must make complete sense and fit with all those involved.

Context and Contracting

The process of change model emphasizes the context for the crisis, including language, culture, gender, personal resources, and more. All of these contextual elements help shape a clear intervention contract, critical to all effective treatment across interventions. This is illustrated in Figure 4.2 and should be kept in mind whenever crisis intervention treatment is initiated.

FIGURE 4.2. The Process of Change Working Diagram of the Therapy Contract

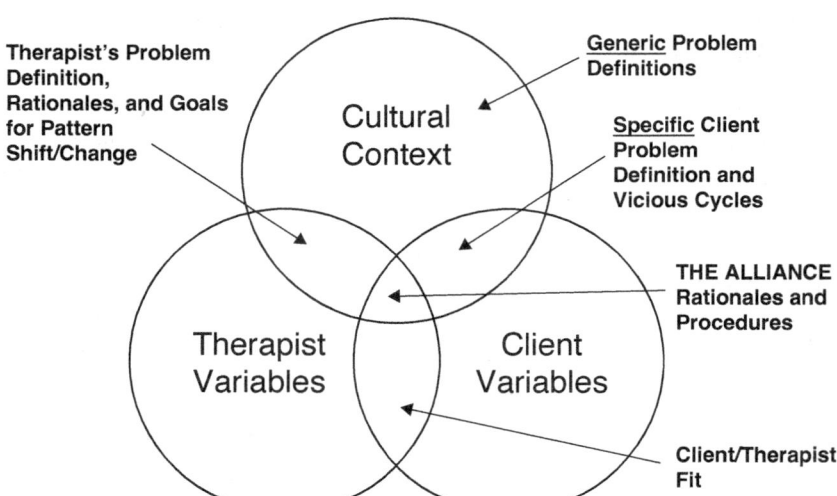

Therapist's Problem Definition, Rationales, and Goals for Pattern Shift/Change

Generic Problem Definitions

Cultural Context

Specific Client Problem Definition and Vicious Cycles

THE ALLIANCE Rationales and Procedures

Therapist Variables

Client Variables

Client/Therapist Fit

The Process of Change Working Diagram of the Therapy Contract

The diagram in Figure 4.2 is the intersection of three spheres. The first is the cultural context shaping how we define what is normal, what we see as problems, and how we are to solve them. The next two spheres represent what therapists and clients bring to the therapy encounter. However, the overlaps or *intersections* of the three deserve particular attention.

First, the overlap of client and culture spheres indicates how the client has both generically and specifically defined their problem, identifies their solutions, and describes subsequent vicious cycles of their solution-generated problem. The client's unique identities and circumstances help to add the specific spin to their problem cycles. Sometimes, the patterns of their problem cycles match those generically prescribed by the culture. Other times, factors specific to the client will alter the specific patterns of their problem.

Second, the intersection of the therapist sphere with the cultural context sphere points to how the therapist's unique multiple identities contribute to their view of the problem and the client through the lens of their particular model of psychotherapy and its related goals. It also implies their target goals for change.

Third, the overlap of the client and therapist spheres indicates how closely the therapist and client's personal characteristics and worldviews match and/or require adaptation to create a good fit between them for a working alliance.

Finally, the *central intersection* of all three spheres represents the nexus of the alliance. The psychotherapy literature generally agrees that the therapeutic alliance is one of the most highly associated components with client change (cf. Norcross, 2002). This includes the typical agreement on a rationale to explain the problem and imply a direction and tasks toward resolution. It also includes the metaconstructions of pattern shift in the client's vicious cycle and the target of *second-order change*, or the needed shift or reversal of the client's failing solution patterns.

While there is much more to be said on this process of change model, it offers a time-honored, sound, metaview or alternative paradigm for doing effective crisis intervention and brief therapy. It not only fits the emerging psychotherapy literature on what works in psychotherapy in general, but it also fills the theory vacuum in the literature on doing crisis intervention. We hope to bring this alive more as we apply the process of change model in Part II of this book.

This approach to defining crises and setting contracts for effective crisis intervention is standard in the process of change model. However, as we will see, this is not always the case in more traditional approaches. In each chapter of Part II, we will also address the cultural context sphere as it shapes the crisis and its responses, and we will note efforts to change that cultural context in the endemic crises of interpersonal partner violence and sexual assault. Now, a final element of the model concerns general interventions that are found and repeatedly applied in the process of change model as it is applied across a wide range of crises.

GENERIC INTERVENTION OPTIONS

Finally, before we move into Part II and address different crises, it will be helpful to lay out several generic intervention options found across the succeeding crisis types. These options include using rationales and reframing (including acknowledging context and contracting within a rationale), normalizing, predicting, positioning and restraining, and prescribing. Each of these general intervention options helps clients make what often feel like risky shifts toward ideas and actions that appear paradoxical or counterintuitive from their current worldview. Often some of these generic interventions stand alone and essentially shape the new direction out of clients' vicious cycles. More often, several of these generic interventions are used in combination to achieve the desired path out of the vortex of each crisis. A brief description of each generic intervention will help to locate them in the next chapters covering each successive type of crisis.

Rationales and Reframing

A strong argument has been made in the general literature on effective psychotherapy that all effective psychotherapies share the process perspective as they help clients break and reverse vicious cycles (Fraser, 2018; Fraser & Solovey, 2007b). In his classic review of psychotherapy and healing traditions, Jerome Frank concluded that all successful therapy involves a trusting relationship, in a healing setting, and a *rationale* or *myth* that guides related procedures (Frank & Frank, 1991).

It is important to note that Frank and Frank (1991) were clear that treatment rationales do not need to be scientifically valid to be effective. The key is that both the clinician and the client believe in them. This idea is supported in Wampold's meta-analysis of psychotherapy outcomes (Wampold, 2001; Wampold & Imel, 2015). Frank's contextual model of treatment describes a two-step process that is crucial to intervening across all approaches to treatment, in which the practitioner first provides an explanation or rationale for the client's symptoms. Then the practitioner offers a procedure designed to change the way that the client is trying to solve the problem. This process coincides with the operational definition of *hope* offered by Snyder et al. (1999). They suggested that clients gain hope when offered an explanation or frame that makes sense of their problem, implies a direction toward resolution, offers procedures to follow toward resolution, and enlists client motivation to go that way.

As we have demonstrated thus far, most effective interventions in crisis appear paradoxical and require some form of frame or rationale for them to make sense to clients so they may follow them. Thus, rationales and frames will be noted over and again as we discuss effective interventions for each different crisis. Rationales and frames for effective interventions across all crises are always used to help clients make sense of doing something new, or even not doing what they have been doing and simply accepting the situation as something not to be fixed or that will resolve on its own.

Reframing is sometimes closely related to rationale. *Reframing* offers an alternate description of a current action, situation, person, or role that fits the facts of a situation as well or better than former frameworks. It may be used on its own or along with another message or directive to shape a new action or thought. Reframing, as we will see, occurs in most interventions across various crises reviewed in Part II. Reframing rigidly held beliefs or ideas on the nature of a crisis and how to resolve it is often the watershed point from which new patterns flow. We will see reframing constantly as we review each new crisis and its related effective interventions.

Normalizing

Normalizing is closely related to rationales, frames, and context. In short, *normalizing* is the term used for placing a person or group's situation and responses in the context of normal response patterns, given the nature of the crisis in its context. This is classically seen in the stage and phase descriptions of grief (although we will discuss critiques of these as we address grief and mourning in Chapter 7). Normalizing is broadly applicable, however, to all the crises we will soon discuss. People in crisis, whether developmental or incidental, have usually not encountered this type of situation before and are less aware of the range of emotions and actions commonly involved within their context. Normalizing, at times, may be the only intervention needed. It may stop clients' repeated attempts to resolve a crisis that may not be one after all. At those times, clients are urged to accept the perceived challenge as a normal phase or transition. This is why it is important for practitioners to stay up to date on the literature on each crisis yet be open to learning the unique traditions and context surrounding their clients. In conjunction with practitioners validating clients' distress and pain, normalizing is often taken as an affirming message that the client is not alone in their experience.

Positioning and Restraining

Positioning and restraining are also somewhat related to one another. They both are defined in relationship to the positions and sense of urgency of all parties involved in each crisis. They both also are done to deliberately shift the interaction patterns of those involved.

Positioning is when the practitioner deliberately adopts a stance often nearly opposite to that taken by the client and helpful others. Clients, for example, typically feel out of control and disempowered in the face of a crisis. Helpful others typically offer suggestions and encouragement, which can paradoxically reaffirm the person's lack of strength and control. In such situations, positioning can take the form of a *one-down position* for the practitioner. For example, often this takes the form of a general statement such as, "Given your situation, and all that you've been through, I'm amazed that you are doing as well as you are." This position tends to be experienced as empowering and a welcome relief. As we will see, this approach is particularly helpful with clients who are suicidal. Often helpful others make attempts to "cheer them up" and offer new options or assure them that things can't really be all that bad. These attempts are usually met with further depression, alienation, or even anger. The suicidal person gets sucked into a pattern where they often feel denied, misunderstood, and even more hopeless. Taking an opposite position and marveling at a person's strength and resilience, or marveling that they are still alive and sharing their distress with the practitioner, draws the person into doing a positive scan to recognize their strengths. This one-down position is often experienced as empathic and begins setting the groundwork for some new possibilities. The same is often done as practitioners admire the courage of a domestic violence survivor. Positioning is frequently an implicit element of many of the interventions we will review in Part II of this book.

Restraining is a form of positioning that seems contradictory to the traditional role of a practitioner, yet it is helpful in many ways. First, when clients in crisis are anxious that an intervenor will quickly press them to take new and unfamiliar steps, hearing a practitioner tell them that they may need to take this slowly to determine the right path is often a relief. Restraints may also draw out clients' motivation for change rather than have that motivation rest in the practitioner's hands. If clients argue that they need to take more immediate action, then this urgency remains in their hands rather than in those of the practitioner. There may also be, for example, very real needs for caution—such as when a survivor in a domestic dispute is considering leaving, as research points to leaving as one of the higher-risk times for women in such relationships (Walker, 2009). This is a point for realistic restraints. Restraints also offer clients and therapists time to deliberate and plan out a safe path if leaving is to be chosen. And there are several more instances where we will see restraints applied in the crises coming up.

Prescribing

Prescribing is evident across most all effective interventions in crisis. Most often it involves prescribing something opposite of what the client in crisis has tried. We will soon see examples with grief and mourning, in which clients trying to "remember to forget" their lost loved one and move on are told to "remember to remember" by setting aside times to recall the loss and grieve in their own way to bring the loved one back into their life. As we will see in Chapter 7 on grief and mourning, one of the newest supported complicated grief interventions prescribes oscillating or alternating days and times to engage in loss-oriented and restoration-oriented activities. Several PTSD treatment approaches ask clients to deliberately reexperience the trauma, write it down and rehearse it, and so on. These and other prescriptions are always embedded in a rationale or a set of frames to help the counterintuitive reversals make sense. Furthermore, quite often upon successful resolution, clients are told to see whether they can go back to their former patterns and reactions. Aside from the difficulty of spontaneously reexperiencing and redoing old patterns and finding that they just cannot regress instantly, this has another advantage. If the client can go back, then this time it is under their control and it can be discussed before moving forward. These prescriptions relate to what is often termed *relapse prevention*.

Predicting

Predicting goes hand in hand with normalizing and contextualizing. *Predicting* is used widely to help those in crisis avoid catastrophizing around anticipated next phases of the crisis for themselves as well as in the response of others, whether they happen to be officials, family members, or friends. This will be seen in our discussion of domestic abuse cycles, grief and mourning, sexual assault, and more. Predicting is used, in essence, to divert future distress and reactions from precipitating a new crisis cycle, while offering a sense of control to all involved. Furthermore, following successful intervention, predicting future challenges may often prevent clients from catastrophizing over new events that may be anticipated yet do not necessarily constitute a crisis.

All of the aforementioned intervention options merge into guidelines for doing the process of change model we will follow through Part II across a wide range of different crises.

FOLLOWING THE PROCESS

Once more it will be useful to lay out the key elements of the process of change model as we have followed the doing of the model:

- There is always a context and history within which each crisis develops.

- All crises begin with a kick point, trigger, or tipping point shift or difference that is viewed as dangerous and likely to threaten those involved.

- There is always a reaction targeting resolution of the perceived crisis by all those involved and shaped by their common life patterns, context, and history.

- There is an inevitable response to the solution attempts, sometimes resulting in resolution or assimilation of the perceived crisis event, yet often evolving into ongoing vicious cycles. Sometimes these vicious cycles resemble common generic patterns around the crisis according to the literature on the problem, yet they may vary with specific differences in the history, culture, or other unique aspects of those involved.

- There are always goals for resolving each crisis by all involved, and these goals need to be identified and collaborated on between practitioners and involved others.

- The network of significant others involved around the perceived crisis always needs to be identified and their positions and responses to the crisis considered as they contribute to the vicious cycles of the crisis or as they may aid in its resolution.

- Interventions inevitably target pattern shifts and reversals in the escalating vicious cycles.

- There is always a need to accept, respect, and utilize the views, values, strengths, and resources of those involved around the perceived crisis.

- Successful interventions always affirm the distress and embrace the goals and values of all involved as they turn the patterns around the crises to interdict and redirect vicious cycles. When evidence-supported interventions are used, they are always adapted and fit the parties involved.

- Once a small pattern shift begins, then it is supported, amplified, and generalized and the success is attributed to those involved rather than the practitioner.

- Phases of the six-step process of change model are relationship establishment, information gathering, consensual problem formation and goal setting, break/recess, problem solving and interventions, and summary and closure.

- The process of change working diagram of the therapy contract includes three domains (the cultural context, the practitioner's domain, and the client's domain), along with their intersections, and must always be kept in mind.

- Generic intervention options include developing rationales and reframing for the crisis (acknowledging context and contracting within a rationale), normalizing, predicting, positioning and restraining, and prescribing.

PART **II** TIPPING POINT
INTERVENTIONS
ACROSS CRISES:
FOLLOWING THE
PROCESS OF
CHANGE MODEL

INTRODUCTION: TIPPING POINT INTERVENTIONS ACROSS CRISES: FOLLOWING THE PROCESS OF CHANGE MODEL

The Chinese Characters for Tipping Points, *Jī Zhì*

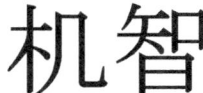

In Part I of this book, we covered a lot of ground in describing the essence of the process of change perspective as it guides crisis intervention. First, we visited a critique of traditional approaches to the idea of crises and doing crisis intervention. We showed how although traditional approaches have served us well in many ways, they have often fallen short. Traditional approaches have relied on inappropriate models of systems and change. In doing so, they have at times missed opportunities for rapid resolutions; at other times, they have even unknowingly fed into the crises they have sought to resolve. We introduced a process model of systems and change and followed its history and main concepts as a more appropriate basis for understanding (a) the human systems we are addressing and (b) the nature of crises and guiding potentially more rapid intervention and resolutions around those crisis points. Chapters 1–3 served as a basis for how to view crises from the process of change model, and Chapter 4 demonstrated how to do crisis intervention from the process of change model.

Our discussion in Part I laid the foundation for this book and culminated in what might be described as a metamodel for viewing and doing crisis intervention across all crises. The Chinese characters, *jī zhì*, that open Part II build on those we presented in the Preface and Part I and symbolize *tipping points*. That is, *jī zhì* translates to being quick-witted or resourceful, symbolizing wisdom. When the characters are combined, *agility* refers to a turning point, *quickness* and *resourcefulness* refer to a turning point, and *wisdom* represents making the kind of wise choices at a tipping point that turn the dangers of crisis into opportunities. As we now transition to Part II, we will follow what are a set of tipping point interventions as viewed through the process of change model as it unifies approaches to crisis intervention across a selected range of different crises (Chapters 5–9). We will address the definitions in the literature of each crisis, follow the patterns found in each one, and look at the interventions recommended and found effective in each case at the respective tipping points of intervention with practitioners. As we do, we will also link each review to the process of change model and note how the literature and recommendations around each separate crisis match the lens of the process view. Finally, we will follow this same format through each successive crisis to show how they all connect and thus guide our work across all crisis intervention and brief therapy. In Chapter 10, we will summarize the work and look to how it guides future practice. We turn first to trauma (Chapter 5) as a paradigm case example of a response to crisis that often cuts across many other crises. We then follow with a sample of incidental, developmental, and endemic crises as we discuss suicide (Chapter 6), grief and mourning (Chapter 7), intimate partner violence (Chapter 8), and sexual assault (Chapter 9). Each chapter in Part II ends with a section called Following the Process (as in Part I), which reviews the essence of each crisis, describes the path of the process of change within it, offers guidelines for the practitioner, and attends to potential secondary stress and trauma of practitioners and how to address it. Although these crises by no means represent the full range of potential crises to be encountered by practitioners, they will be offered as templates to apply moving forward.

5

TRAUMA

Stress, Disorder, and Growth

All crises are stressful by definition. Some crises are traumatic. Thankfully, most survivors either assimilate or accommodate their lives following crises and traumatic events. Some, however, develop posttraumatic stress disorder (PTSD); others move toward posttraumatic growth (PTG). Yet, what makes the difference between developing ongoing disorder or growth? Is there a tipping point that we can identify, and is there a process to follow that might help shape the nature of that future trajectory from negative to neutral or even positive? A look at the literature on trauma may help with that answer.

First, consider the following case of the Taylor family.[1] We will revisit this case at the end of the chapter to demonstrate successful intervention through the process of change model, further noting how the literature on treating PTSD converges on that intervention.

The Taylor family experienced a traumatic event 2 weeks before they contacted a therapist. Late one night, Mr. and Mrs. Taylor awoke to find a shadowy figure in their bedroom going through their drawers. When Mr. Taylor asked

---

[1]All case examples are based on real clients, whose identities have been disguised to maintain confidentiality.

https://doi.org/10.1037/0000445-006
Crisis Intervention: Using Tipping Points to Achieve Transformative Change in Therapy, by J. S. Fraser

who it was, the intruder showed a gun. The intruder demanded that the couple lie on their stomachs and then wanted to know where their money and jewelry were. He told Mr. and Mrs. Taylor not to cry out or he would hurt their son in the next room. Both heard the intruder yank the landline telephone off the wall and pull the phone cords off, and they feared he was planning to use the cords to bind them. Ms. Taylor was unaware of the intruder's gun until it went off. Not knowing that the shot was accidental and sure that her husband had been killed, a strange, detached sense of calm overtook Ms. Taylor as she thought, "So this is how it ends . . . execution style . . . first him and now me." This thought was broken by the reassuring movement of her husband and then by the sinking realization that their 17-year-old son, Dan, had been awakened by the shot and entered their bedroom. When the burglar demanded that Dan lie face down between his parents, their terror peaked again. Suddenly, the voice again told them not to call for help. They heard footsteps on the stairs and the front door slam. The burglar was gone.

When Ms. Taylor called for an appointment for therapy 2 weeks later, she had not been able to sleep more than a few hours a night since the break-in. She was constantly fearful, especially of the dark, and she was unable to concentrate at work. Mr. Taylor had been taking care of both the police reports and insurance details while he stayed up most nights with his wife. He was throwing himself into home and work projects, yet his attention was becoming scattered and diffused as his exhaustion increased. Their son, aggravated by his parents' response and frustrated by newly locked doors and windows and by a new burglar alarm, was engaging in escalating arguments with his parents, especially his mother.

This case is just one example of a traumatic event impacting a whole family, yet affecting each family member in a different way as they sought to recover. This example is similar in some ways yet different from a set of traumatic responses discussed in an earlier publication (Fraser & Solovey, 2007b). There, we recounted the cases of a 70-year-old survivor with recurring night terrors from his battlefield experience in World War I, and a devout Jewish father in Tel Aviv who could not shake the recurrent flashbacks of a teenaged girl's severed head under a park bench following a bombing. In Chapter 4 of this volume, we discussed the case of Ann, a young woman who had vivid recurring dreams and hallucinations of men taunting her following a sexual assault. These cases were all resolved through intervention, yet in different ways: The World War I survivor's night terrors stopped after he told his fascinated stepson about them. The devout Jewish father's flashbacks stopped after he underwent a procedure referred to as eye movement desensitization and reprocessing (EMDR), in which he repeatedly imagined the terrible image while tracking a finger moving back and forth. Finally, after Ann's therapist validated her distress over the sexual assault, Ann stopped having dreams and hallucinations in which men taunted and degraded her; she then agreed not to dispute the dreams and hallucinations and moved forward with her life. Each of these interventions was different, yet each resolution converged on rather similar forms.

This chapter will thus add to what we know about trauma and treating PTSD and will include what we have learned about PTG. In that process, we will also look at how such traumatic tipping points might be shaped in more desired new directions. First, we will define trauma and posttraumatic stress, then we will address PTG. Next, we will turn to the commonalities present in effective PTSD interventions and what we have learned of the process of PTG. Finally, we will return to the case of the Taylors and follow how the process of change model was used to turn the entire family away from their trauma-escalating responses and toward them all moving forward with their lives.

TRAUMA AND POSTTRAUMA

We turn first to definitions of PTSD from the dominant Western culture source, the *Diagnostic and Statistical Manual of Mental Disorders, Fifth Edition* (*DSM-5*; American Psychiatric Association, 2013). Whereas PTSD was classified as an anxiety disorder in previous *DSM* editions, the *DSM-5* describes PTSD as a trauma- and stressor-related problem, accounting for the common range of emotions beyond anxiety (e.g., anger, sadness, guilt, or horror) and alternations in thoughts and mood. The *International Statistical Classification of Diseases and Related Health Problems, Tenth Revision* (*ICD-10*; World Health Organization, 2017), mirrors this shift yet includes three variations of PTSD: unspecified, acute, and chronic.

The first major criterion for PTSD, differing from other disorders, requires the person to have experienced, witnessed, or otherwise faced an event or events involving actual or threatened death, serious injury, or sexual violence from which the person does not recover emotionally, behaviorally, or both (American Psychiatric Association, 2013). Symptoms cluster into categories of reexperiencing, avoiding, negative alterations in cognition and mood (e.g., memory difficulties, feeling detached, or persistent negative beliefs), and hyperarousal.

- *Reexperiencing* may include memories of the trauma coming up without warning, vivid flashbacks of intense reexperiencing the trauma, nightmares of the event, or experiencing intense terror, disgust, sadness, rapid breathing, or heart rate triggered by cues similar to the traumatic event.

- *Avoidance symptoms* include avoiding thoughts and feelings about the trauma, situations and events similar to the trauma, and related intense feelings associated with them. Paradoxically, temporary relief from decreasing painful emotions typically increases avoidance patterns in the classic vicious cycles in anxiety and depression.

- *Negative alterations in cognitions and mood* often include detachment or numbing to reduce painful feelings from intrusive memories, yet some survivors experience the opposite by having continuous intense emotions such as anger or shame. This category also includes cognitive symptoms such as self-blame, the idea that person will never be normal again, or that nowhere is safe.

- *Hyperarousal* is similar to the person being in a constant fight-or-flight state as they may have been during the traumatic event. Hyperarousal may include constant scanning for danger cues and constant states of tension eventually resulting in sleep disturbances, irritability, overreactions, and decreased concentration.

Because many, if not most, of these symptoms are present for most people who have experienced intense traumatic events, several criteria must be met for PTSD to be diagnosed. These criteria are as follows (American Psychiatric Association, 2013):

- The symptoms must have been experienced for at least a month following the event.

- At least one intrusion example must be present, such as recurrent dreams, distressing memories, and physiological responses to trauma cues.

- Avoidance of either internal or external reminders of the traumatic event is also required.

- The person also must be experiencing at least two of the following symptoms: forgetting important parts of the traumatic event; exaggerated negative thoughts about oneself, others, or the world; distorted blame of oneself or others; detachment or estrangement from others; inability to experience positive emotions; lack of interest in activities; or globally negative experiences of fear, horror, anger, guilt, or shame.

Prevalence

PTSD is relatively prevalent. Except for specific phobias and social phobia, PTSD exceeds all anxiety disorders in prevalence (Kessler et al., 2005). In a prevalence study of U.S. civilians, Kessler et al. found that 20.4% of women and 8.2% of men were likely to develop PTSD following trauma experiences. Rape was identified as most likely to lead to PTSD in both men and women. For men, the probability of PTSD following other events was 39% for those exposed in combat, 24% for those who experienced childhood neglect, and 22% for those who experienced physical abuse in childhood. For women, the prevalence of PTSD from traumatic events other than rape was 49% for those who had experienced childhood physical abuse, 33% for those who had been threatened with a weapon, 27% for those who had been sexually molested, and 21% for those who had been physically attacked. Accidents and natural disasters showed much less likelihood of producing PTSD.

There has been a convergence of agreement that generally five broad phases tend to occur as people recover from traumatic events (Figley, 1988):

- First is the emergency or outcry phase, with heightened arousal and fight-or-flight responses.

- Second is the emotional numbing and denial phase, including avoiding and numbing from the experience.

- Third is the intrusive-repetitive phase, including intrusive thoughts and images and rumination over the incident and how to integrate it.

- Fourth is the reflective-transition phase, including coming more to grips with the trauma and putting it into a larger personal perspective either positively or negatively.

- Last is the integration phase, in which success involves successful integration of the trauma into the person's life and new worldview.

Exactly how each survivor moves through these phases will shape their eventual lifepath toward resolution or posttraumatic stress or growth.

POSTTRAUMATIC STRESS DISORDER MODELS

Four major models have been put forward over the years to explain the process of PTSD, including alternatives from learning theory, information processing theory, cognitive theories, and constructivist theories.

Learning Theory

Early on, learning theory views of PTSD were based on the Mowrer (1960) two-factor theory, combining classical and operational conditioning. Intense distress from a traumatic event was said to be associated with stimuli related to the traumatic event and setting. Then, when the conditioned memory or other related cues of the event elicit fear and other intense emotions, people's escape and avoidance responses reduce intense emotions and become operationally reinforced to occur again with greater frequency. This prevents the link between the trauma cues from extinguishing despite the absence of the original danger. The vicious cycle becomes self-perpetuating. However, this learning theory had trouble explaining the occurrence of repetitive intrusive traumatic memories and nightmares.

Information Processing Theory

Lang (1977) proposed that a fear network develops in memory that triggers escape and avoidance. The fear network includes stimuli, response, and meaning components comprising a schema, or a fear structure elicited by anything associated with the traumatic event. This fear structure is proposed to be reactivated relatively frequently in people experiencing PTSD. When activated, the full package of the fear network reenters consciousness, causing intrusive memories and flashbacks. Subsequent attempts to avoid this reactivation account for the avoidance symptoms of PTSD. The solution-generated process evolves.

Cognitive Theories

Similar to information processing theory, cognitive theories turn their focus on the survivor's belief system, addressing how the person adjusts their prior beliefs and expectations to the traumatic event. Without being fully integrated into existing beliefs and expectations, memories and trauma-associated stimuli retain their ability to trigger intrusive and avoidant reactions. In some ways, this is similar to the Piagetian concepts of assimilation and accommodation to novel events. A dynamic tension is thought to arise, creating swings between the need to integrate the experience on the one hand and the need to avoid the emotional pain arising from intrusive thoughts and trauma-related stimuli on the other hand. This vacillating cycle sustains and amplifies PTSD. Ehlers and Clark (2000) proposed that people with PTSD are unable to see the event as time-limited and generalize it to the future. Assuming that normal events are more dangerous than they are, people with PTSD overestimate the probability that the traumatic event will recur. They see false alarms as true alarms or see their symptoms as signs they cannot cope with similar threats in the future. Still others propose alternate two-stage theories (Brewin et al., 1996) that memories consist of

(a) those that are nonconscious and not easily accessed and (b) those that are verbally accessible and may be called up voluntarily. The first memories may be triggered by cues similar to the trauma or deliberate thoughts of the trauma and result in intense intrusive sensory images or flashbacks and intense physiological arousal; the second memories consist of cognitive appraisals of the event. The first memories produce conditioned emotions of fear and anger; the second memories yield secondary emotions that add guilt, shame, and sadness. The first memory pattern is said to be best treated by exposure therapy, whereas the second is suggested to be best treated by cognitive behavior therapy. However, no matter which approach is used, the intervention reverses the pattern of avoidance.

Constructivist Theories

Turning to the content of cognitions around the traumatic event, constructivist views address how the traumatic event shatters survivors' basic assumptions about a safe world. Their prior beliefs about safety, trust, predictability, control, esteem, and intimacy, to name a few, are violated by the traumatic event. Resick et al. (2016) used the "just world" myth to explain how traumatic events destroy the human wish for a predictable and controllable world. Survivors' natural avoidance of intense emotions, as well as the uncontrollability and unpredictability created by memories and trauma-related stimuli, thus inhibits the event from being fully assimilated into their beliefs and expectations. From a constructivist perspective, however, the person's prior beliefs and appraisals will also shape their reactions to the perceived threat of the trauma. Fearing that reexperiencing emotion may overwhelm them, many survivors will avoid thoughts about the event and stay busy as much as they can. Others may feel they need to make sense of the event and ruminate about how it happened and how to prevent it. Still others may become immobilized and have trouble making decisions, feeling that the event was punishment in some way for something they did. This view postulates alternate response patterns for alternate points of view. Recall the Venn diagram of the process model (Figure 4.2, this volume). These individual differences reflect unique elements from the client sphere, creating variations in the resulting vicious cycles. Nevertheless, the solution once more creates and perpetuates the problem.

Physiologically Based Theories

A more recent trend has focused attention on the physiological bases of trauma and posttrauma. Bessel van der Kolk's (2014) *The Body Keeps the Score* focused on the long-lasting physiological imprint of trauma. As of this writing, the book has spent 280 weeks on the *New York Times* paperback nonfiction best-seller list and has been translated into 37 languages. In essence, van der Kolk argued that trauma is a special type of memory that embeds permanently in the brain and may resurface unbidden long after the traumatic event is over. For one reason or another, the popularity of *The Body Keeps the Score* has transformed the cultural lexicon to define nearly every stressful experience as a trauma (incorrectly, of course). van der Kolk rejects this popularization of his work, yet he stands by the position that trauma stays embedded in our physiology until it is adequately released in a supportive environment (Carr, 2023). However, van der Kolk's crusade in advocating and conducting workshops on his perspective has made a mark on the popular culture more recently. For example, Carr (2023) recently published a *New York Magazine* article, "Trauma: America's Favorite Diagnosis," with the subtitle, "Tell Me Why It Hurts: How Bessel van der Kolk's Once Controversial Theory of Trauma Became the Dominant Way We Make Sense of Our Lives," suggesting an almost faddish growth in the theory's popularity.

Vicious Cycles of Posttraumatic Stress Disorder

Recall the process of change paradigm of open, dynamic, self-organizing systems discussed in Part I of this volume. The first premise is that systems are ever changing and constantly evolving in an alternating spiral of negative and positive feedback processes. Those processes are constrained by the context of the system (as in the riverbanks and river bottom of Heraclitus' river and the language and cultural contexts discussed in Chapter 2). As in Gregory Bateson's (1979) evolutionary spiral, attempts at stability at one level (or negative feedback) will spiral into positive feedback to the next level, where increased stabilizing efforts will likely feed into the next escalation, and so on. Following the social constructionist view, if the system neither assimilates nor accommodates new input needing attention, then the new input is likely to serve as a trigger for escalating vicious cycles. Regarding context and following the work of Bateson, not all differences or new inputs into a system will trigger a response. As Bateson (1978) said, the input must be "a difference that makes a difference" in the context of the system (p. 453). For some individuals or in some cultures, a given event may be experienced as normal, as expected, or as more of the same, and the system takes little note. However, for others, the same event or change may draw intense attention and response. The process perspective on change suggests that all such failures at assimilation or accommodation will fuel a pattern of escalating cycles of positive feedback, or *vicious cycles*. Peoples' attempts to assimilate or accommodate the experienced traumatic event while dealing with its accompanying intense emotions often succeed following an interval of adjustment. Some individuals may not even experience the same event as traumatic within their own worldview or personal or cultural context. However, failed attempts to assimilate or accommodate intense and traumatic events such as death (actual, witnessed, or threatened), serious injury, or sexual violence will likely trigger escalating vicious cycles fitting the symptoms of PTSD.

All of the aforementioned theories of PTSD suggest that the survivors of trauma find themselves trapped in vicious cycles similar to the mastery by avoidance patterns seen with anxiety and depression. Another trap is survivors' attempts to remember to forget the trauma and its emotions, resulting in the event and its emotions surfacing at unexpected times or places or in dreams. As usual, these patterns each have different bases for their explanation. As we will soon find out, most evidence-supported approaches to treatment target mastery by avoidance and remembering-to-forget patterns, and their interventions do just that—that is, they have the survivor reverse and go toward the distressing experience and habituate, assimilate, or accommodate it in one way or another. This retains the now familiar counterintuitive paradox of second-order change as clients get out of the child's finger trap, so to speak, by pushing in and going toward their dilemma rather than pulling away. They must go toward the trauma rather than away to move beyond it. They must remember to remember to escape the paradox of their past solutions.

Another perspective on the solution patterns of trauma survivors experiencing PTSD is that they remain overly engaged with the event, while at the same time overlooking its impact and not taking new and different directions to move forward. As we will also see, some newer, present-centered approaches to PTSD have been found as equally effective as those that focus on variations of exposure. These present-centered approaches help clients acknowledge the traumatic event and its distress, then collaborate to redirect their efforts to present and future solutions. This intervention essentially blocks and redirects prior vicious cycles, reorienting clients toward present and future directions. This is an alternative second-order pattern reversal to that of exposure treatments. Furthermore, these present-centered approaches have the added benefit of engaging many clients with PTSD in treatment who simply cannot face the paradoxical solution of reexperiencing their trauma and its intense emotions through exposure-based approaches.

As we have seen from the process view, the bottom lines in all psychotherapies that work are helping clients interdict and reverse their problem-generating solution patterns, or the vicious cycles of their problem. To do this, all approaches engender felt validation and trust in clients to step out of the level of their current solution-generated problems and enter into a metalevel working alliance with their therapist. From this metalevel, clients can view the failed solution patterns surrounding their problem, accept a new and fitting frame for their problem, and buy into a related treatment rationale that helps make sense of new and formerly counterintuitive solutions (cf. Fraser, 2018; Fraser & Solovey, 2007a, 2007b). This same pattern recurs across all evidence-supported approaches to PTSD.

TREATMENTS THAT WORK FOR PTSD

Turning to treatments that work for PTSD, the first stop might be the website for research-supported psychological treatments for PTSD, compiled by the Society of Clinical Psychology (Division 12 of the American Psychological Association [APA]). Seven treatments are listed: five are strongly supported, one has modest research support, and one (psychological debriefing) has no support and is considered potentially harmful (American Psychological Association, 2022). Of the five strongly supported treatments, three are considered exposure-based approaches and two as present-centered or combination approaches. The strongly supported exposure-based treatments include prolonged exposure (PE; for overviews, see Foa et al., 2018; McLean & Foa, 2011), cognitive processing therapy (CPT; for summaries and reviews, see Resick et al., 2016, 2024), and EMDR (Shapiro, 2012, 2017). The two present-based approaches are present-centered therapy (PCT) and stress inoculation training, with strong and modest support, respectively. For the purposes of this chapter, all of the strongly supported approaches will be discussed.

Exposure-Based Approaches

As noted earlier, given the vicious cycles of mastery by avoidance evident in the descriptions of PTSD, the logical intervention involves reversing those patterns and exposing clients to their traumatic experiences and emotions. This paradoxical intervention from the perspective of survivors requires not only a trusting and supportive treatment alliance with the therapist but also problem frames and treatment rationales that help clients make sense of doing the opposite of what seems logical to them. As with depression (Fraser, 2018), several of these approaches use different premises and problem frames to help clients with this process. PE has a behavioral base, CPT has an obvious cognitive base, and EMDR is based on the effect of rapid eye movement. Interestingly, the biologically based explanation of van der Kolk (2014) recommends using a range of exposure approaches such as PE and EMDR, rather than turning to medication options for treatment (see also Interlandi, 2014). Rather than further detailing each of these approaches here, it may be most useful for our purposes to turn to another alternative approach that does not emphasize exposure to see how it fits with our process of change perspective.[2] Next, we discuss PCT.

Present-Centered Therapy

Given how much sense it makes to have survivors who actively avoid trauma to reverse their solution pattern and go toward the experience to master it, it seems to make little sense to do anything else. However, researchers have found PCT to be equally effective (Frost et al., 2014). An interesting point is that this result came almost by accident. In attempting to devise more bona fide yet nonspecific treatments to use in clinical trials testing the specific effects of different therapy approaches to PTSD, a present-focused alternative was designed that avoided exposure to past trauma. McDonagh et al. (2005) described PCT as follows:

> It is a collaborative therapeutic intervention in which the therapist's informa-tion and expertise are used to assist the client to recognize the impact of her trauma history on her present coping style and by teaching her a systematic approach to problem solving to enhance coping. The main elements of PCT are psychoeducation about the diagnosis of PTSD and the common aftereffects of childhood trauma, training in problem solving, and journal writing . . . PCT was specifically designed to omit the hypothesized active ingredients of CBT (breathing retraining, PE, in vivo exposure, and CR). Although the role of trauma was acknowledged in assessing current difficulties, the trauma itself was never the focus of the treatment. (p. 518)

No present-centered approach used in research employs exposure. In fact, it is assiduously avoided at all costs. However, PCT has been found comparable enough to current strongly effective approaches to PTSD to be included in the APA Division 12 list of evidence-supported treatments (American Psy-chological Association, 2022).

How does PCT fit with the process of change view? As stated earlier, present-centered approaches acknowledge the traumatic event and its distress, then collaborate to redirect the survivor's efforts to present and future solutions. This intervention essentially blocks and redirects prior vicious cycles, reori-enting clients toward present and future directions. This is an alternative second-order pattern reversal to that of exposure treatments. Instead of

---

[2]For a further summary of each of these exposure-based approaches, the reader is referred to Fraser (2018, Chapter 8 on PTSD, pp. 177–184).

clients being overly engaged in struggling with or avoiding past traumatic events (or both), their attention is reversed and redirected to present and future effective problem solving and interpersonal effectiveness. This pattern redirection from former vicious cycles makes perfect sense as a resolution to former solution-generated patterns of over involvement with the past and the trauma. Furthermore, these present-centered approaches have the added benefit of engaging many clients with PTSD in treatment who simply cannot face the paradoxical solution of reexperiencing their trauma and its intense emotions through exposure-based approaches. The dropout rate for PCT has been found to be significantly less than exposure-based approaches (Imel et al., 2013).

To this point on dropouts, a meta-analysis of dropout in treatments for PTSD found little difference in dropout rates across most active treatments, with the exception of PCT (Imel et al., 2013). Across three large trials, including 695 patients in total, the dropout rate was lower for PCT compared with trauma-specific treatments. Imel et al. concluded by saying,

> if future research replicates this pattern of comparative efficacy and a lower rate of dropout relative to other treatment modalities, it would seem appropriate to consider PCT a first line treatment, especially for patients who do not prefer a trauma-focused treatment. (p. 402)

With regard to dropout rates from PTSD treatments, Benish et al. (2008) concluded the following:

> Due to the fact that about one-quarter of patients drop out of psychotherapy treatment for PTSD (Hembree et al., 2003) and dropout appears to be related to symptom change (Bradley et al., 2005), keeping patients in treatment would appear to be more important in achieving desired outcomes than would prescribing a particular type of psychotherapy. Having several psychotherapies to choose from may enable a better match of patients to type of psychotherapy that fits the patient's worldview and is more tolerable to that particular patient. (pp. 755–756)

These conclusions match those from the psychotherapy literature reviewed in Part I (this volume), which recommend flexibility on the part of therapists and fitting approaches to client preferences rather than prescribing a one-size-fits-all approach. This may be especially true when working with clients with PTSD who may be, quite understandably, very reluctant to go toward or reexperience their trauma. Clearly, many clients develop the kind of trust in their therapist and belief in the frame for their problem and its related treatment rationale, such that they are able to devote themselves to the paradoxical task of immersing themselves in the trauma they have struggled so long to avoid. However, as we can now see in the PCT alternative, others can be helped equally well by not having to do so—and yet still make the pattern reversal needed by devoting their efforts and attention to their present and future effectiveness rather than staying mired in their past trauma. This all fits perfectly with the process paradigm. Many paths may lead to the same results, as we saw in the discussion of the open process system concept of equifinality in Part I.

POSTTRAUMATIC GROWTH AS AN ALTERNATIVE

Although our discussion of trauma and treatments for posttraumatic stress is encouraging, our original points from Part I of this book emphasize that crises and crisis intervention have traditionally focused on the potential damage invariably resulting in the wake of crises. It is undeniable that a great number of people are drawn into the vortex of PTSD following traumatic events; more survivors clearly either assimilate or accommodate to experienced traumas, and others actually show signs of growth and even thriving in their lives posttrauma. As mentioned at the beginning of this chapter, a process view of open human systems views crises—in particular, traumatic events—as potential *tipping points*. Depending on the context, perspectives, and reactions of all involved at these critical junctions, future paths for those involved may vary from what may be judged as neutral, distressed, or genuinely positive. We turn now to the findings on what has come to be called posttraumatic growth or PTG.

Growth as an Alternative

In their classic work, Tedeschi and Calhoun (1996) first coined the term *posttraumatic growth*, referring to the phenomenon then being noticed in the literature that a significant number of people actually experience positive outcomes following traumatic events. They described this in a summary article as follows:

> Posttraumatic growth describes the experience of individuals whose development, at least in some areas, has surpassed what was present before the struggle with crises occurred. The individual has not only survived, but has experienced changes that are viewed as important, and that go beyond what was the previous status quo. Posttraumatic growth is not simply a return to baseline—it is an experience of improvement that for some persons is deeply profound . . . Posttraumatic growth, then, has a quality of transformation, or a qualitative change in functioning, unlike the apparently similar concepts of resilience, sense of coherence, optimism, and hardness. (Tedeschi & Calhoun, 2004b, p. 4)

The Posttraumatic Growth Inventory (Tedeschi & Calhoun, 1996) measures five domains of growth, which have been adopted as standard across studies of the concept. These domains include the following:

- greater appreciation of life and changed sense of priorities;
- warmer, more intimate relationships with others;
- a greater sense of personal strength;
- recognition of new possibilities or paths for one's life; and
- spiritual development.

Describing these five domains, Tedeschi and Calhoun (1996) said, "Each of the five domains of posttraumatic growth tends to have a paradoxical element to it that represents a special case of the general paradox of this field: that out of loss there is gain" (p. 6). They concluded that many people facing trauma actually experience growth from their struggle. It is the process of struggle following the event that is critical to the eventual positive or negative trajectory. Although a traumatic event is never desirable, the good that comes out of the process of having to struggle with it is what defines potential growth. This could not be a better validation for our earlier discussion of chaos theory, cusps, and essential tipping points in open social systems. It is not the nature of the trigger or the traumatic crisis point that determines the outcome; it is the context and process that follows that determines future positive or negative paths.

Violating Our Assumptive World

As we discussed in Part I, crises—in particular, traumatic ones—often present stark challenges to our assumptive worlds where most all of us assume life is relatively safe, ordered, predictable, and manageable. When we are confronted with challenges to our just and stable world assumptions, we are challenged to either assimilate or accommodate our worldviews to the reality presented by the crisis or traumatic event. These have been referred to as "shattered assumptions" and relate to shattered assumption theory (Janoff-Bulman, 2010; Schuler & Boals, 2016). Greater levels of threat to our core beliefs have been found to be associated with higher levels of posttraumatic stress (Cann et al., 2010). As we noted earlier, sometimes (really oftentimes), people's efforts are successful in adapting to traumatic events and they move forward, informed now that crises do occur, yet they are still moving within relatively similar views of their world. Alternatively, the process of struggling with the aftermath of a traumatic event or crisis may lead to ongoing or even relatively permanent distress or centrally defining their life around the occurrence of the traumatic event.

Aldwin, Carver, and colleagues have done classic work using dynamical systems concepts to describe how new patterns of functioning can emerge from the process of adapting to crises that present discrepancies from our assumptive worldviews (Aldwin, 2009; Carver & Scheier, 1982, 2000; Rasmussen et al., 2006). In essence, they suggested that individual differences in coping abilities, process of coping, and point of view differentiate between some people who set upon a maladaptive vicious cycle and others who proceed on an adaptive positive feedback cycle. Carver and Scheier (1982, 2000) suggested that often some early success in coping tips the process toward PTG, and the centrality and importance of the events to one's core beliefs determines how strongly people struggle for resolution versus giving up. Tedeschi and Calhoun (2004b) found that those who report growth after trauma often need to disengage, or give up, prior assumptions while persisting in building new schemas, goals, and meanings. No matter what, however, all trauma is distressing. While typical patterns immediately following traumatic events are cognitive and emotionally numbing and in the near term intrusive recollections of the event, intrusive negative rumination is typically frequent. Eventually, if the process of recovery is effective, people disengage more from the event and adjust to a new life pattern in the wake of the experience. Nearly everyone who reports PTG, however, also reports experiencing at least some distress (Tedeschi & Calhoun, 2004b). People experiencing less distress or who come to more rapid resolution are those for whom the trauma has been more easily assimilated or accommodated within their experienced worldview. There is less struggle. Some ongoing distress may actually be important to the process of struggling toward some form of resolution. The key to the positive or negative trajectory posttrauma appears to lie in the nature of the process of the struggle for resolution.

Searching for Meaning

Relating to issues of grief, loss, and mourning, Neimeyer (2000, 2001) emphasized the nearly universal quest to make meaning of our losses. Our context, culture, language, and values help to shape that process. How important or central to our core beliefs the traumatic event is viewed to be also helps shape the nature of that search. Groleau et al. (2013) suggested that the research finds two kinds of rumination—intrusive and deliberate. *Intrusive rumination* occurs when not intended; *deliberative rumination* occurs when the individual deliberately tries to gain perspective and meaning on the traumatic event and its aftermath. Based on their work and a review of the literature, Cann et al. (2010) concluded that deliberate rumination was positively related to PTG, whereas intrusive rumination was strongly related to PTSD.

The focus thus becomes how survivors search for meaning following trauma. The literature notes that both distressing and positive elements are always present following any traumatic event. This leads us to the conclusion that it is the way survivors struggle with finding meaning that shapes their course. In this way, what emerges is the potential for practitioners to follow a dual-process model of intervention similar to that discussed in a grief and mourning intervention by Stroebe and Schut and described in Chapter 7 on grief in this volume (Richardson, 2010; Schut, 1999; Stroebe & Schut, 2001a, 2008, 2010). In this model, clients are offered validation, time, and space to experience the intrusive and painful elements of their traumatic experience deliberately, and then alternate that with a more planful and deliberate perspective-taking time to reflect on how the trauma will fit into their life going forward. Critical to this and all effective treatment is to have this occur in a validating, supportive, and warm environment both socially and in treatment. In fact, this is exactly what occurs in all of the effective treatments covered earlier.

Positively Resolving Crises and Trauma

The literature suggests that clinicians may want to attend to the adaptive rebuilding of their clients' assumptive world (Janoff-Bulman, 2010). In addressing culturally competent practices in supporting PTG around the world, Weiss and Berger (2010) suggested that clinicians may need to help survivors rebuild an understanding of themselves and their place in the world, which is both adaptive and aware of the many ways in which individual worldviews vary across cultures. As noted earlier, deliberate rumination or processing of trauma is highly correlated with PTG (Cann et al., 2010; Groleau et al., 2013; Tedeschi & Calhoun, 2004b). Conversely, *negative repeated rumination* is strongly associated with distress and deterioration. The literature shows that both the seeds of deterioration and growth coexist in traumatic experiences across all 10 cultures studied (Taku et al., 2021). It is how the survivor addresses that Escher-like picture such that when viewed one way, the viewer sees white geese over a dark terrain; when viewed another way, the viewer sees dark geese flying over a light ground. Whether viewed either positively or negatively, that tends to initiate the ongoing process from there. These same authors addressed the paradoxical nature of trauma as a *both–and phenomenon* rather than viewing deterioration and growth as independent, dichotomous outcomes.

Maercker and Zoellner (2004) proposed the concept of the Janus face model conceiving of PTG as having an *illusory* side and a *constructive* side. Describing the illusory side, they pointed to findings that some survivors and those around them often decide to directly emphasize the positive elements of a traumatic event without struggling more deliberately to sort it out and come to a more transformative resolution. In that illusory case, these survivors tend to use that quickly concluded optimistic conclusion as a way to mask and deny the distress of the trauma at present and in the long run. It is only through a more deliberate, constructive, and planful struggle with the distress of trauma that survivors tend to evolve more transformative worldviews that both account for the distress of the trauma and evolve new goals and directions to move forward. Janoff-Bulman (2004) stated the following:

> Strength through suffering, psychological preparedness, and existential reevaluations involve confrontations with agonizing challenges and painful realizations. The positive and negative are inextricably linked. The long-term legacy of trauma involves both losses and gains. As in the case of reversible figures, the survivor can focus on one or the other, but both are ever present. (p. 34)

Tedeschi and Calhoun (2004b) stated that

> Psychological crisis can be defined in relation to the extent to which the fundamental components of the assumptive world are challenged, including assumptions about the benevolence, predictability, and controllability of the world; one's safety is challenged, and one's identity and future are challenged. (p. 5; see also Janoff-Bulman, 2010)

The individual's growth evolves exclusively with confrontation with the distress of the trauma. The individual needs to engage with cognitive processing to generate a new narrative from their shattered assumptive world in order to emerge with growth. The process is what is important to the outcome. How one ruminates or attempts to sort out the aftermath of trauma makes a powerful difference.

Looking at the nature of rumination following traumatic events, Michael et al. (2007) studied PTSD in assault survivors. They found a high incidence of rumination in all survivors with PTSD. However, the occasional occurrence of rumination was not necessarily a sign of PTSD. Instead, it was the nature of ruminations and worry that was linked with the severity of PTSD. In their words, they found the "occurrence of 'why' and 'what if' type questions and unproductive thinking, compulsion to continue ruminating, negative feelings during and after rumination" (p. 314) associated with PTSD. This kind of rumination constituted a form of *emotional avoidance* while often triggering emotional intrusions of the event itself without any positive frame into which they could be understood. This process tended to initiate negative feelings while ruminating and often triggered more intrusive memories, which required more rumination, resulting in the vicious cycles typical of PTSD. Again, it is the way one struggles with the aftermath of trauma that sets the positive or negative direction of resolution, not the traumatic event itself. As described earlier, two types of rumination have been discovered: intrusive rumination often occurs as an automatic uncontrollable negative thought, whereas deliberate rumination is more effortful, constructive, and intentional in nature. Thus, confronting the disconfirmation of one's assumed safe assumptive world with a planned and deliberate process is strongly associated with developing a transformed new understanding of oneself and one's place in the world. Such is the process of change linked with growth.

Disclosure in a Positive Context

Active disclosure of thoughts and emotions to empathetic others may also be important to the development of PTG (Tedeschi & Calhoun, 2004b). In a study of PTG across 10 cultures, Taku et al. (2021) reported,

> One robust finding in the current study is the role of positive disclosure on PTG and negative disclosure on PTD . . . the experience of positive disclosure led to PTG in all countries studied. These findings suggest that the individual experience of PTG may be inseparable from social connections and is likely to be fostered when the person felt relieved and helped after they talked about the event. (p. 4)

On the other hand, when disclosure is met with blame, aversion, or restraint and thus received negatively, there is strong correlation with avoidance, shame, and negative self-images associated with PTSD.

Zoellner and Maercker (2006) stated that

> Psychotherapy constitutes a good context to explore positive changes in the aftermath of trauma. The simultaneous acknowledgement of patients' suffering enables them—on the basis of a trustful and intimate therapeutic relationship— to explore positive changes as a result of their coping process as well. (p. 650)

In addition, Zoellner and Maercker (2006) emphasized the following:

> It seems important to raise clinicians' awareness of the possibility of growth. Only then are they able to perceive PTG, as their clients begin to consider such possibilities. For too long clinicians may have short-changed trauma survivors by focusing so closely on reducing symptoms of trauma, that they may have failed to support clients as they reflect upon their basic beliefs more generally . . . A professional abstinence from a naive use of positive thinking should be accompanied by an open-minded attitude on the side of the therapist allowing patients to find their own specific meanings, interpretations, ways of coping and recovery. (p. 650)

A PROCESS OF CHANGE APPROACH TO CRISES AND TRAUMA

This is the essence of what we are discussing as a process of change model of crises and crisis intervention. All effective approaches to psychotherapy (a) establish a supportive, trusting relationship; (b) offer a mutually acceptable and flexible rationale to understand the nature of the problem and to make sense to clients of the often paradoxical pattern shifts needed for resolution; and (c) then support that process and reflection as the intervention evolves (Fraser, 1995c, 1998b, 2001; Fraser & Solovey, 2007b). Across all crises, resolution converges on similar, often counterintuitive pattern shifts and reversals. The process of helping clients understand such often paradoxical tasks and comply with them comes down to the concepts of *flexibility* and *fit*. Practitioners need to be flexible in their choice among sometimes equally effective approaches (to trauma, in the present case). As we have seen, each approach may be based on different premises and explanations for the trauma as well as the related rationales and procedures for treatment. For example, PE, CPT, and EMDR, along with PCT, are all judged to work equally well. Fitting them to what the survivor may accept and understand and what the practitioner believes will be helpful is what is meant by flexibility on the part of the practitioner and fit with clients or survivors.

As we have seen through exploring how some survivors of trauma have grasped the opportunity of crisis to grow through pain, it emphasizes what we see in many of these effective approaches to PTSD. Each offers a rationale for the trauma according to their own view. Each develops a supporting, trusting context for disclosure and treatment. In addition, each prescribes a deliberate process of reexperiencing that pain on the one hand, then deliberately developing their own sense of meaning and a new understanding of their life and goals moving forward while acknowledging the occurrence of the trauma, often the loss, and anguish of the event on the other hand. Even the present-centered alternative, which diligently does not prescribe that the survivor reexperience their trauma, offers an acceptable rationale to understand the trauma and its effects, validates the trauma as indeed distressing, and then prescribes very deliberate processes of integrating the trauma into their own current life context and develops goals and pathways for the future. All of these effective approaches, in fact, match with what we have found out about what works in the process of PTG.

As we discussed in Part I, the nature of what those involved with crises do as they engage in the tipping point of a crisis will determine whether the danger or opportunity of each crisis will emerge. As we will see with each successive section of Part II, as practitioners learn the generic patterns within what is known of each crisis, as well as what has been found to be effective in intervention, they will begin to master a process of change perspective on how to support the opportunity of each new crisis with their clients and those around them.

Applying the Process of Change Model

As promised at the beginning of this chapter, we now return to the case of the Taylor family. Recall that the family had been traumatized by a burglar who had broken into their home, lined them up face-down on a bed, had a gun that fired inadvertently, and then fled the home. Ms. Taylor was the main person requesting help from the therapist, yet both her husband and son were still reacting to the break-in in problematic ways.

The Risks of the Current Patterns

The current solutions of all the family members hold a series of potential escalating risks. Ms. Taylor may begin a cycle of self-doubt and fear, which might lead to chronic insomnia, phobias, family alienation, social isolation, or job loss, among other possibilities. Other family members may come to see and treat her as somehow altered, sick, or bad, as opposed to her formerly capable and engaging self. Mr. Taylor may gradually build resentment over his wife's fears and begin to alienate himself from her through either withdrawal or gradual escalation of arguments over her irrational fears. He also may succumb to exhaustion, physical illness, or job loss. Their son's increasing frustration and arguments with his mother might not only lead to reinforcement of his mother's sick role or his father's stress cycle (or both), but they also may increase his alienation from his parents and contribute to generalized disputes in other areas of family life or social interaction.

The family's contact with the therapist offered another potential tipping point to interdict and redirect these vicious cycle reactions and turn them toward a new, safer, and fulfilling future. The key was to intervene quickly and intensely with each and all members of the family and meet with them often during the window of opportunity offered by their openness and motivation to move beyond the sequelae of the break-in. The pattern of interventions with the family offers a nice window into the phases of process of change intervention, including collaboration with the family around their goals, interventions, and results of the process of change model. We turn now to highlight each phase.

Tracing the Process of Change Intervention Phases

The practice of the staff within the hospital-based crisis and brief therapy center where the intervention was carried out was to meet with clients within 24 to 48 hours of their first request for service unless they walked in or presented to the hospital emergency room, when they would be seen immediately by available practitioners on staff. Then, up to 10 sessions could be flexibly scheduled to address the presenting complaints and then allow for gradual spacing of sessions and check-ins in the future. Recall that the process of change intervention model has six phases that parallel and converge on both best practices for most all effective psychotherapy (cf. Barlow, 2021; Norcross, 2011) and, in this case, include a convergence of interventions recommended throughout this chapter in treating and resolving trauma. These phases are as follows: (a) establishing the relationship; (b) gathering information on the problem and the response patterns surrounding it; (c) reaching consensus on the problem, along with goals and a rationale for moving forward; (d) taking a brief break either within the session or pausing briefly for a consultation with a colleague; (e) active problem solving, including in-session interventions, homework, and a plan for follow-up; and (f) providing a summary of the session, with reinforcement and enlistment of clients' values, strengths, and goals and a reiteration of the plan with follow-up sessions laid out, and upon success, inoculation against falling back into the same patterns as new distressing events or triggers occur.

Following these phases through the intervention with the Taylors will further bring the model to light to show how the practitioner assessed the vicious cycle patterns; aligned with the strengths, perspectives, values, and goals of each member; developed a rationale for reversing those patterns and making sense of prior counterintuitive actions; supported shifts as they occurred; and, finally, congratulated everyone on their successes and strengths. We will take each phase separately and highlight it with each family member as follows.

Establishing the relationship. Ms. Taylor was seen first alone, and the practitioner validated her distress, given the break-in and the fact that the intruder had not been caught and other break-ins had occurred in the neighborhood. After two sessions, Mr. Taylor was seen alone and the practitioner validated his concern for his wife, along with his exhaustion over needing to take care of her and all involved with things going forward. The son was soon also seen on his own, and the practitioner affirmed his frustration with everything following the break-in, as well as his wish for his mother to regain her grasp on her life and that of the family.

Gathering information on the problem and response patterns surrounding it. The practitioner learned that Ms. Taylor had always been a strong leader in the home and in her job as an administrator for a local political leader. Since the break-in, Ms. Taylor found herself startling at the least noise and dissolving in tears as she recalled the terror or the break-in when trying to make her husband and son understand all of that. She had tried to suppress the memory of that terror, yet it would again come to mind when she least expected it. She was also worried about falling asleep for fear of recurrent nightmares. She also recounted prior distress in the household when their daughter took the car and ran away with a boyfriend, and when her son showed her his cut wrists after a breakup with a girlfriend. She just felt overwhelmed and had been missing work. Mr. Taylor had thrown himself into building a deck, communicating with the police, installing an alarm system in the home, and reassuring his wife, staying up with her at night until she went to sleep; he had been missing work, as had his wife. The Taylors' son, Dan, came in at the request of the practitioner to offer his view of the problem. He was fed up with dealing with alarms going off, struggling with locked doors, and having to tiptoe around in the morning to get out early to his summer job at a golf course. Dan also found himself arguing with his mother about how she "needed to get over all this stuff." His mother had always been so strong. He could not understand why she was now so weak.

Reaching consensus on the problem, along with goals and a rationale for moving forward. Ms. Taylor simply wanted to stop startling at the least thing, to have her husband and son understand her fears, and to regain her former strength and control at home and work. Mr. Taylor simply wanted the same, and he also wanted to be able to relax and sleep again. Above all, he really just wanted his strong and capable wife back. Their son wanted things back to normal and for his mom to return to her place as a strong doer in the family.

Taking a break to distance. Upon taking a break and gaining some perspective on the vicious cycles evident in the family, the practitioner laid out the following plan. The practitioner planned to have Ms. Taylor reverse her denial and instead spend time on her own remembering the trauma, taking perspective on it, and also writing down her dreams. Mr. Taylor was to begin asking his wife for more advice and help with his projects. Mr. Taylor was also to let his wife know he needed more sleep, so he was going to start turning off the lights and going to sleep on his own as he could. Their son was to tell his mother he understood her stress by relating it to the distress he felt after breaking up with his girlfriend. He was to begin a habit of checking all the doors and windows with his mother at night and waking up his parents each morning to let them know he was leaving.

Active problem solving and interventions. Ms. Taylor agreed that she needed to integrate the aftermath of the break-in more, and she was willing to move toward reexperiencing the images. She was also willing to set aside time to think of what might have happened if her son and husband had been killed and she was to allow herself to cry if she needed to. Before bed at night, she agreed to place a notepad beside the bed to record her dreams if she woke up. The next morning, she would reflect on what she had written. Mr. Taylor agreed that he had been getting in the way of his wife's strengths and needed to allow her to recapture them. He was also quite willing to begin taking a one-down position with her by asking for her advice and help. At night he would let her know he needed sleep and turn out the bedroom lights. Their son thought the practitioner made sense when he said Dan needed to share more with his mom about his pain at breaking up with his girlfriend and tell her he would join her in regaining her strength as he has done himself. In fact, he had always admired his mother's strengths. He agreed to remind her to check the windows and doors each night and volunteered to split the task with her. Each morning, he would let his parents know he was up and about to leave for his golf course job by knocking on their bedroom door and saying he was leaving for the morning.

Summary and follow-up plans. The family was seen a total of six times spaced over about 3 weeks. Each session concluded with a summary of what happened in the session and plans for homework. A final session included the entire family about 6 weeks after the initial visit. Ms. Taylor had found it difficult to recapture the terror when she set time aside to deliberately reexperience it. Surprisingly, those flashbacks to the break-in had diminished so much that they rarely happened. She was also sleeping better with few chances to wake and record her dreams. Best of all, she saw their household returning to normal as she felt closer to her husband and son and returned to work. As Ms. Taylor reversed her solutions of avoiding the trauma and instead embraced the process of going toward it and integrating it into her life, the fear, flashbacks, and nightmares subsided. Furthermore, as her husband reversed his caretaking and protecting efforts with his wife and instead tapped back into her strengths and collaborations, he saw that strength and assurance return to her. As for their son, his morning knocks at the bedroom door helped him stop walking on eggshells and helped his parents get used to normal reasons for awaking to sounds in their bedroom. Another byproduct of the son sharing his recovery from breaking up with his girlfriend, as well as supporting his mother's need to do what she needed to as she recovered herself, was a renewed closeness between mother and son as things returned to normal.

In summary, the whole family (in this case, the problem-generated system) literally reversed their prior problem-generated solutions (those vicious cycle escalating patterns) and rediscovered their joint strengths in the aftermath of intense adversity. A final reflection here is that there was most likely a healing effect of all family members retelling the trauma experience, being validated for their reactions, and having them normalized. Counterintuitive solution reversals were helped to make sense to all through both joint and individual rationales for explaining the distress and implying that the opposite paths would lead to reintegrating the experience and resetting their future paths. The final full family session was spent first by the practitioner positioning with the family through admiring the family's strengths and resilience. Discovering that the break-in was on Mr. Taylor's birthday, the practitioner predicted everyone being reminded next year of the event, and they all laughed over planning a break-in anniversary party next year. All were inoculated against overreaction at future challenges by the reminder that "life is a roller coaster" and there would be more normal and unexpected challenges down the road, yet they had all discovered their individual and joint strengths to move through each new hurdle as a result of how well they had done overcoming this one.

FOLLOWING THE PROCESS

Following the process view of trauma, PTSD, and potential PTG helps us see how effective interventions across specific approaches converge on a very similar pattern of interrupting and reversing vicious cycle solutions. Retracing the literature, we find the following:

- No event is traumatic in itself. It is the way the event is viewed and reacted to that determines the subsequent path toward resolution, PTSD, or eventual growth.

- Practitioners should acknowledge the cultural context of the trauma and how it is understood, track solution patterns to identify vicious cycles, then validate the distress and fit a rationale for understanding it and either prescribe exposure or redirect new actions toward resolution (often alternating between both).

- The most common distress patterns in traumatic distress involve mastery by avoidance. Thus, most effective interventions revolve around rationales supporting exposure. Even a present-centered approach serves to interdict the vicious cycle solution cycles by redirecting attention and efforts from trying to master the trauma through avoidance (and getting caught in the vicious cycle of needing to remember the trauma over and again to try to forget it) to instead striving for valued goals in the future.

- While there are several equally effective approaches to PTSD, they all involve fitting an accepted rationale for understanding the distress and enlisting either exposure to aid assimilation or redirecting actions to future resolution while validating the distress.

- Clearly, interdicting repeated attention and vicious cycle–focused solutions around crises may also be achieved by acknowledging the distress yet building on people's values and goals to redirect their efforts toward present strengths and future plans and directions as in the present-centered options now found to be equally helpful.

- Interventions should always build on strengths and enlist support networks for support and reinforcement of the treatment rationale and process, as seen with the case of the Taylor family.

- Along with building on strengths, it is always important to build narratives in the direction of growth and transformation, if possible, as practitioners acknowledge the intensity of the trauma while taking positions identifying and admiring people's strengths in the face of adversity. This in itself is a reversal at a larger level from treating trauma as an inevitable tipping point for PTSD and instead redirecting attention to its potential for introducing transformative change and growth.

- Finally, as noted initially, most all of these elements dealing with trauma will be found across the wide range of different crises, as we will discover in the coming chapters on suicide, grief and mourning, intimate partner violence, and sexual assault, among other variations.

6

SUICIDAL CRISES

Hazardous Intersections

Consider this often-quoted statement by a woman in a suicide survivors' group that echoed the sentiment of the group: "We could only have talked to a person who we knew would not be afraid of listening, without judging. In a suicidal crisis we could never have trusted a person who would want to talk us out of it" (Michel & Jobes, 2011, pp. 5–6).

This chapter will trace the parallel patterns for people who are potentially suicidal and the typical intervention patterns of practitioners (for better and worse) as we lay out how the process of change view fits the trajectory of individuals contemplating suicide and matches interventions recommended to be effective. For practitioners facing the tipping point of a suicidal crisis, there is great pressure to intervene. As noted in a now classic work by Chiles and Strosahl (1995),

> There are at least two widely accepted assumptions that create this pressure: 1) there are specific factors that foretell suicidal behavior in a given individual (i.e., risk factors), and 2) there is a correct intervention (either medication or crisis intervention) that will prevent the behavior from occurring. Unfortunately, there is very little research that supports either of these ideas. (p. 35)

https://doi.org/10.1037/0000445-007
Crisis Intervention: Using Tipping Points to Achieve Transformative Change in Therapy, by J. S. Fraser

This pressure, of course, is compounded by the growing incidents of lawsuits claiming malpractice around completed suicides, the demands of managed care to practice only evidence-based approaches, and the trends toward rapid diagnosis, rapid-acting medication, and short hospitalizations. Practitioners are naturally drawn into the threat-rigidity cycle discussed in Part I, in which their focus narrows and they attend rigidly to a simple goal of managing risks and decreasing liability. Just as with most suicidal clients, under a sense of agitation and urgency to resolve the presenting crisis, practitioners and helpful others are drawn into the vicious cycle of increasingly conservative actions, rejection of outside input and alternatives, and a mechanized shift into rigid, black-and-white thinking.

Such direct attempts to stop others from suicide reflect what we discussed as first-order change that makes sense yet makes things worse and is better resolved by interventions fitting the category of second-order change, which make things better yet does not often make sense in emergencies (Watzlawick et al., 1974). Another example is Daniel Kahneman's (2011) Systems 1 and 2 thinking, in which tried-and-true reactions typically get locked in during a crisis even though they make things worse. This follows the threat-rigidity hypothesis as well (Staw et al., 1981). Most often, direct efforts to try and focus on risk or talk someone out of suicide tend to backfire. Yet what are we to do when we encounter someone seriously considering killing themselves? This chapter endeavors to answer that question by making apparently counterintuitive yet effective suicide interventions make sense in the face of the literature and through related rationales to help practitioners tip their clients away from suicide and instead toward achieving their values and goals. We will begin by looking into what we have learned about understanding and predicting suicidal intent, and then step into what we have found to be most effective in averting and redirecting it.

PREDICTING SUICIDE

Suicide is the paradigm case of a crisis. After all, it represents the potential end of a life! So much has been written on suicide that its discussion could easily take over the remainder of this book and still fall short. However, suicide is also a low base-rate phenomenon. What this means is that there are many people who fit the risk profiles for suicide who do not eventually contemplate or attempt suicide; these risk factors are merely normative averages and cannot be used to predict an individual's behavior. Regarding this, Chiles and Strosahl (1995) said,

The assumption that suicide can be predicted is a myth in search of some facts . . . Although many mental health professionals presume that an important clinical skill is the ability to assess the imminent risk of suicide, this capacity has never been empirically demonstrated. The algebra for such predictive abilities is just not there. Partly, this is a base rate problem because, fortunately, suicide is a rare event. Suicide risk factors are useful in identifying high-risk *groups*, but they are much less useful in identifying high risk *individuals*. (pp. 7–8, emphasis in original)

. . . thinking about suicide is extremely common in the general population, whereas completed suicide is extremely rare. Practically speaking, it means that thinking or talking about suicide is not really an accurate predictor of attempting suicide in the next 24–48 hours. (p. 36)

We discussed this earlier as we reviewed the nature of the open systems and of dynamical process-based systems and their tipping points through chaos and catastrophe theory analyses. Each case in some way will follow its own unique pathway. An eventual trigger or perturbation to push an individual to attempting suicide may or may not occur.

Yet statistics on suicide cannot be overlooked. World Health Organization data for 2019 estimated that 703,000 people die by suicide each year worldwide; in addition, an estimated 1 in every 100 deaths are by suicide, the global suicide rate is over twice as high for men than women, over half of all suicidal deaths occur before age 50 years, and suicide is the fourth leading cause of death in 15- to 29-year-olds (World Health Organization, 2021). As of February 2023, suicide rates in the United States climbed again after a 2-year decline, with an increase of 30% (adjusted for age) between 2000 and 2020 (Dhungel et al., 2023). In response to these trends, the National Suicide Prevention Lifeline in the US changed its name to 988 Suicide and Crisis Lifeline (https://988lifeline.org/) in July 2022, as part of a national attempt to increase access to help.

Greater access to mental health resources is undeniably needed and a positive step. However, turning again to how such tipping points can best foster the opportunity of crises in the dangerous opportunity equation, the nature of the intersection between a person contemplating suicide and their practitioner on the other end of the line or in the emergency room is what is most important. As stated earlier, helpers may either help or hinder in a crisis. There is no single effective approach to intervening successfully with suicide. Regarding this dilemma, it has been said, "For instance, we know a lot about personal and clinical risk factors for suicide. However, in spite of a vast literature on suicide risk factors, predicting future suicidal behavior and being able to anticipate when to intervene are virtually impossible" (Michel & Jobes, 2011, p. 4).

Nevertheless, when viewed from the process of change, there is a core process of how most suicidal crises evolve and how the basic draw of their potential danger often escalates the suicidal cycle. Finally, following the same process thread, there are nearly universal intervention processes leading to resolution. Yet what seems to be universal around suicidal intent?

PSYCHACHE AND TIPPING POINTS

Edwin Shneidman and Norman Farberow might be said to be two of the parents of suicide intervention through their early work with the Los Angeles Suicide Prevention Center (Farberow & Shneidman, 1961; Shneidman & Farberow, 1965). While Emile Durkheim (2005) stands out as maybe the most prominent theorist from a sociological perspective, Shneidman has likely contributed the most to sorting out triggers for suicide that fill most of the lists of risk factors.

Shneidman, the founder of suicidology, coined the term *psychache* as a key part of his cubic model of suicide (1993). This term is meant to capture the intolerable psychological pain preceding suicide, and Shneidman (1993) suggested that it is the one variable that relates to all suicides. The cubic model combines dimensions of psychache (intolerable psychological pain), perturbation (or the degree of disturbance or agitation), and press (or the buildup of multiple stress factors creating urgency), which, as they all converge, create the eventual probability of suicide. This model thus focuses on the process evolution of an individual eventually reaching the tipping point to kill themselves, mirroring the dynamical systems concepts of movement within a system toward the chaos and sudden catastrophic shifts discussed in Part I.

Regarding the most common characteristics of those who complete suicide, Shneidman (1985) listed 10 convergent factors:

1. The common purpose of suicide is to seek a solution.
2. The common goal of suicide is the cessation of consciousness.
3. The common stimulus is psychological pain.
4. The common stressor is frustrated psychological needs.
5. The common emotions are hopelessness and helplessness.
6. The common internal attitude toward suicide is ambivalence.
7. The common cognitive state is constriction of thinking and choices.
8. The common action is toward escape.
9. The common interpersonal act is often communication of intention.
10. The common consistency in suicide is often lifelong problematic coping patterns.

These categories circumvent the common lists of combined risk factors of elements such as age, race, gender, and so on.

In their interpersonal approach, Joiner et al. (2009) combined three other factors emphasizing interpersonal relationships. The first is a decreasing fear of death and pain, thus *acquiring suicidal capability*. The second is *perceived burdensomeness* to others. The third is a lack of attachment or value to others, or *failed belongingness*. This view also suggests that a gradual buildup of all three at once is necessary to reach the critical threshold of suicide. Again, it reflects the same overall idea of the process of change model in moving key factors most salient in one's context to an eventual tipping point. This view mirrors the gradual buildup to all-or-nothing changes or cliffs in open systems as viewed from our discussion of chaos theory and catastrophes in Part I. Recall our discussion (Chapter 2) of Heraclitus's river moving through sudden shifts as the force of the flow increased, moving suddenly to new vicious cycle whirlpools and on to unpredictable chaos.

Through their description of the *three I's*, Chiles and Strosahl (1995) offered perhaps one of the simplest convergent approaches to understanding when people increase their potential for suicide beyond applying simple risk lists. They suggested the following:

> Any person has the potential to become suicidal when confronted with a situation that produces emotional pain *and* is believed to be *inescapable, interminable,* and *intolerable* (i.e., the Three I's). When the person believes that no effort will be sufficient to solve the problem, it becomes inescapable. When there is no expectation that the situation will change of its own accord if it is not somehow solved, the problem becomes interminable. When the individual cannot tolerate the amount of emotional pain that the situation is producing, the problem is intolerable. (p. 60, emphasis in original)

A strong element of this perspective is that it places the person and their view and capabilities in the context of their situation and at the center of focus for the practitioner. Once more, the emphasis is on an evolving process to an eventual trigger point that is different for each individual. (This is reminiscent of Konrad Lorenz's (2021) illustration of the fight-or-flight impulse in dogs discussed earlier in Chapter 2 relating to catastrophe theory, in which just one critical factor will tip the dog over a cliff to either attack or flee.)

SUICIDE AS NOT A "THING IN ITSELF"

With apologies to Immanuel Kant, suicide is not a "thing in itself" (Cholbi, 2010). It does not exist as a thing out of context or a problem or pathology on its own to be cured or solved. Instead, suicide is a potential solution to a perceived problem considered inescapable, interminable, and intolerable, as Chiles and Strosahl (1995) put it. Bryan (2021) suggested that the reason suicide rates have remained stubbornly high for decades is the outdated notion that mental illness is what causes suicide. Bryan said,

> We have decades of research that, that core assumption—the bedrock of prevention efforts nowadays—is wrong. Because we've thought of suicide as a mental health problem—something inside people—we say—You suffer from depression and need to go to treatment . . . but therapy and medications won't pay your bills, won't help you have a boss who treats you with dignity and respect, won't change the neighborhood you're in. (Clay, 2023, pp. 3–4)

Similarly, in the introduction to *Building a Therapeutic Alliance With the Suicidal Patient*, Michel and Jobes (2011) stated,

> *Suicidal behavior* is not a psychiatric diagnosis, such as depression or schizophrenia, but it is an act (or action) that always has its very personal and individual inner truth. Studies that evaluate therapies for suicidal patients have taught us that it is notoriously difficult to provide evidence that we can effectively reduce the risk of suicidal behavior, including death by suicide. (p. 3, emphasis in the original)

Suicide is a response to a perceived intolerable and painful situation that seems hopeless to change. When viewed as an option in the face of an intolerable and interminable situation, suicide becomes a reasonable option that might be considered as a client and practitioner evaluate other potential solutions to the problem at hand. Most professional training either implicitly or explicitly teaches most practitioners to avoid any risk of potential suicide and to focus all efforts on preventing it. However, suicidal individuals are best served by acknowledging their pain and collaborating in a problem-solving alliance to address the dilemma that is feeding that pain. This is the essence of the entire volume by Michel and Jobes (2011) on building empathy and a therapeutic alliance with people feeling suicidal. It is also a key element of several intervention models we will cover in this chapter. Managing suicidal risk rather than treating it as a disorder is the convergent pathway in the literature more recently (cf. Chiles & Strosahl, 1995; Joiner et al., 2009; Michel & Jobes, 2011).

RISK-ORIENTED VERSUS TREATMENT-ORIENTED ASSESSMENTS

Chiles and Strosahl (1995) offered a concise contrast between a risk-oriented assessment versus a treatment-oriented assessment, according to key issues as follows. Risk management positions are presented first and then compared with treatment-oriented positions second.

1. *Session focus*—Risk-oriented assessment aims to assess and manage risk; treatment-oriented assessment reframes suicidality as problem solving.

2. *Knowing suicide risk factors*—Risk-oriented assessment considers this knowledge a central and very important part of interaction; treatment-oriented assessment considers it less important, as it is collected in the problem-solving context.

3. *The importance of assigning a reliable risk level*—Risk-oriented assessment considers the reliable risk level central to treatment; treatment-oriented assessment considers it less important, as suicide potential is not predictable.

4. *Risk management concerns*—Risk-oriented assessment has a very high focus on risk factors, with preparation to take strong steps to protect patients; treatment-oriented assessment has a low focus on risk factors because suicidal behavior per se cannot be prevented, and it instead turns to the person's pressing problems.

5. *Stance regarding ongoing suicidal behavior*—Risk-oriented assessment has a prohibitive focus on ongoing detection and prevention; treatment-oriented assessment anticipates the stance and uses it to collect data about ongoing problem solving.

6. *Legitimacy of suicidal behavior*—Risk-oriented assessment considers suicidal behavior as a problem to be gotten rid of; treatment-oriented assessment considers suicidal behavior as a legitimate but costly form of problem solving.

7. *Time allotted for discussing suicidality*—Risk-oriented assessment devotes much more session time to discussing suicidality; treatment-oriented assessment devotes much less session time to such discussion.

8. *Prevention orientation*—In risk-oriented assessment, most strategies are built around preventing suicidal behavior; treatment-oriented assessment uses fewer prevention strategies and places more focus on problem resolution strategies.

These assessments are also summarized in Table 6.1.

THE PROBLEM WITH NO-SUICIDE CONTRACTS

Most practitioners and most service agencies have so-called no-suicide contracts as a basic risk management component of their protocols for addressing suicidal clients. Typically, a no-suicide contract is a written and signed agreement in which a client agrees not to kill themself for a specific

TABLE 6.1. Comparison of Risk-Oriented Versus Treatment-Oriented Assessments

Key issues	Risk-oriented assessment	Treatment-oriented assessment
Session focus	Assess and manage risk	Reframe suicidality as problem solving
Knowing suicide risk factors	A central and very important part of interaction	Less important, as it is collected in the problem-solving context
Importance of assigning a "reliable risk level"	Central to treatment	Less important as suicide potential is not predictable
Risk management concerns	Very high focus on risk factors with preparation to take strong steps to protect patients	Low focus on risk factors, as suicidal behavior per se cannot be prevented, turning instead to the person's pressing problems
Stance regarding ongoing suicidal behavior	Prohibitive focus on ongoing detection and prevention	Anticipated, and used to collect data about ongoing problem solving
Legitimacy of suicidal behavior	Suicidal behavior is a problem to be eliminated	Suicidal behavior is a legitimate but costly form of problem solving
Time allotted for discussing suicidality	Much more session time	Much less session time
Prevention orientation	Most strategies are built around preventing suicidal behavior	Fewer prevention strategies and more focus on problem resolution strategies

Note. Data from Chiles and Strosahl (1995).

period of time, with specific responsibilities of both the client and the clinician and a contingency plan if a crisis intercedes to jeopardize a client's ability to honor the contract. The problem with the idea of a no-suicide contract is that it focuses on stopping suicide rather than addressing the problems that lead a person to consider suicide. Trying to prevent suicide directly feeds into the vicious cycle created by others opposing suicide, but it also puts the person who is suicidal in the position of defending their personal reasons for suicide.

There are many additional reasons not to resort to directly trying to prevent suicide through no-suicide contracts and otherwise. First, although plans of action are helpful, devising a plan for what a client should do as part of a creative problem-solving plan is preferable to what they promise not to do. M. C. Miller (1999) resonated with these points in his chapter on suicide prevention contracts, making a compelling argument that the idea of a contract is misguided and does more to relieve the liability concerns of clinicians and agencies than it does to prevent suicide. In their article on the case against no-suicide contracts, Rudd et al. (2006) noted that despite more than a dozen studies (which are often methodologically flawed), few have found the contracts to be effective:

> It is difficult to imagine that having known the patient for only a session or two, perhaps even the first time we have met, we would ask the patient to relinquish the right to self-determination, particularly if we have yet actually to provide anything concrete in the treatment exchange, such as symptom relief or the necessary skills for effective self-management. (p. 247)

In reality, suicide is always an option, especially at times of intense psychological pain, and this needs to be affirmed within an ongoing treatment plan to develop a life worth living, as aptly put in the dialectical behavior therapy (DBT) approach of Marsha Linehan (2014). All of the problem-solving approaches to the suicide intervention dilemma (cf. Chiles & Strosahl, 1995; Joiner et al., 2009; Linehan, 2014; Linehan et al., 2015; Michel & Jobes, 2011) advocate for variations of commitment-to-treatment plans that do not restrict a patient's rights with respect to the option of suicide while making a commitment to living. Rudd et al. (2006) defined such commitment-to-treatment contracts as follows:

> It is defined as an agreement between the patient and clinician in which the patient agrees to make a commitment to the treatment process and living by (1) identifying the roles, obligations, and expectations of both the clinician and the patient in treatment; (2) communicating openly and honestly about all aspects of treatment including suicide; and (3) accessing identified emergency services during periods of crisis that might threaten the patient's ability to honor the agreement. (p. 247)

These commitment plans are then combined with crisis response plans: When the client finds themself considering acting on their suicidal thoughts, they identify what is upsetting them, consider a more reasonable set of options, review what they have concluded about what has tended to bring them to suicidal points in the past, and then engage in things that help them feel better for at least 30 minutes. By taking these steps, the person slows down and steps out of the vicious cycle to take perspective on it. If they still have the same intense wish for suicide after completing this exercise, they agree to contact a specific emergency number or go to an identified emergency room. As part of a treatment approach that builds skills and new plans to handle the kind of problems that have led the person to seriously considering ending their life, these commitment-to-treatment and crisis response plans hold much greater promise of actually reducing the probability of suicide than do the popular no-suicide contracts or other treatment plans that aim to directly prevent suicide.

This problem-solving approach fits well with the metaview of the process of change, in that it focuses on the most recent trigger point of the current vicious cycles and directs collaboration toward shifting and redirecting that current vicious cycle. This problem-solving approach also takes advantage of some of the therapy literature's most resounding correlates with positive change in therapy, such as high motivation, clear goal setting, empathy, and a strong therapeutic alliance (Fraser, 1995b, 2001, 2018; Norcross, 2011).

James and Gilliland (2016) reviewed a composite of factors and warning signs from the American Association of Suicidology and other resources. They concluded that whenever four or five of the following factors are present, a crisis worker should consider a person to be at high risk:

> serious suicidal impulses; a family history of suicide; previous attempts; a specific plan; access to lethal means; the recent loss of a loved one; the anniversary of a traumatic loss; a destabilized family around loss, personal abuse, violence, or sexual abuse; is psychotic; is abusing alcohol/drugs; had had a recent trauma; recent unsuccessful medical treatment, chronic pain or terminal illness; lives alone; depressed or recovering from depression or recently released from hospitalization for depression; giving away possessions; earlier episodes of physical, emotional, or sexual abuse; pervasive feelings of hopelessness/helplessness; preoccupied and troubled by earlier trauma; shows profound levels of emotion; threatened financial loss; ideas of persecution; sexual orientation distress; unplanned pregnancy; history of incarceration; dwelling on death and suicide; feeling not missed if gone; and chronic and acute stressors. (pp. 119–120)

PROMISING PATHWAYS TO POSITIVE INTERSECTIONS

If we see suicidal crises as hazardous intersections or tipping points between clients and their context and between therapists and clients, then what might be some more positive intersections for opening new options for better futures? As we have discussed thus far, both clients and helpers are prone to the threat-rigidity cycle of narrowing focus to tunnel vision and all-or-nothing thinking at suicidal crisis points. Figure 4.2 presents the process of change working diagram of the therapy contract that we described in Chapter 4, which may offer the clearest explanation of how four potentially more effective approaches resolve this dilemma (cf. Chiles & Strosahl, 1995; Joiner et al., 2009; Linehan, 2014; Linehan et al., 2015; Michel & Jobes, 2011). Next, we will address each sphere of the diagram in turn and then discuss overlaps and central convergence in the following sections.

The Therapist Sphere

First and foremost, the four current approaches described in this chapter address the most important qualities of therapists as they encounter suicidal crises. Chiles and Strosahl (1995), Joiner et al. (2009), Linehan and colleagues (Linehan, 2014; Linehan et al., 2015), and Michel and Jobes (2011) offered four closely related approaches to effective suicide intervention. Each of these four major approaches to suicide intervention addresses therapist attitudes and anxieties when confronting suicidal clients. One edited text, for instance, is devoted entirely to chapters on building a therapeutic alliance with the suicidal patient, emphasizing it as an essential prerequisite for any intervention with suicidal patients (Michel & Jobes, 2011). They all do this to counteract the intense and natural tendency for all helpers—practitioners, in particular—to get drawn into the vortex of pure risk management as they converge on similar profiles for effective practitioners.

In his clinical assessment and management of suicide (CAMS) approach, Jobes (2016) offered diagrams contrasting the problematic one-up approach, in which the practitioner is in charge, with the more collaborative side-by-side relationship of practitioner and client. Chiles and Strosahl (1995) devoted an entire chapter to examining the affective, ethical, and legal issues of a practitioner contracting collaboratively with clients in order to counteract becoming drawn into an emotional vortex with them. Chiles and Strosahl suggested the following: being "matter of fact" with the suicidal patient; "normalizing" suicidal behavior as legitimate in the current context; validating the client's sense of pain; setting a collaborative set with the patient by framing suicidal behavior as problem-solving behavior; and forming a short-term action plan to evaluate suicidal feelings and weigh alternative choices and set positive goals (p. 79). Linehan's DBT approach to chronically suicidal patients advocates that therapists not only offer a casual and relaxed approach to the idea of suicide, but they also use radical acceptance and validation of the person in the face of their overwhelming pain and their desire to kill themselves (Linehan, 2014; Linehan et al., 2015). The clinician becomes a clinical problem-solver to build distress tolerance and new interpersonal skills. In the conclusions to *Building a Therapeutic Alliance With the Suicidal Patient*, Michel and Jobes (2011) stated,

> First and foremost, we believe in a patient-oriented approach; the patients are the experts of their suicidal struggle, and the clinician's job is to find a way to walk along with patients on their idiosyncratic suicidal trail. . . . We also clearly believe in the primacy of the therapeutic alliance as the essential vehicle for traveling along with the suicidal patient. (p. 380)

All of these current positions address the intersection with clients in our process of change working diagram of the therapy contract (Figure 4.2) by reversing the traditional one-up risk finding and risk prevention position with the practitioner in charge and taking a knowing stance. Instead, it advocates a one-down validating and collaborating stance in which the practitioner is a learner and listener to the client considering suicide, which is counterintuitive from a traditional view yet now judged as a more effective path.

The Client Sphere

Dovetailing with the aforementioned approaches to clients considering suicide are a set of important ways of viewing these clients. These approaches include understanding the major characteristics and normative aspects of most clients considering suicide. Yet more importantly, they include (a) viewing these clients as responding to an important distressing problem serving as a trigger point tipping them toward suicide and (b) acknowledging the downward spiral of growing tunnel views of life as well as black-and-white, all-or-none thinking and growing desperation through the threat-rigidity cycle. All emphasize the idea of slowing down decision making, contracting to evaluate alternatives, increasing tolerance for distress, and decreasing at least one or more of the three I's (inescapable, interminable, and intolerable) put forward by Chiles and Strosahl (1995). All approaches engage in positive goal setting, increasing hope, and increasing positive social connections to replace feelings of alienation and burden to others. This addresses the overlaps with both the therapist and cultural spheres of the process of change working diagram of the therapy contract (Figure 4.2).

The Cultural Sphere

Once again, all of these approaches consider culture by addressing the nature of the culture's religious beliefs about suicide, governmental prohibitions against suicide, and sanctions following completion for survivors. These approaches also consider the nature of gender rules and definitions of appropriate and desirable roles and behavior. These get translated into personal and cultural "shoulds" or expected roles and behaviors for members of the culture, resulting in personal feelings of shame and guilt and appraisals of failure. All authors of the four approaches described in this chapter address social networks to the extent that they offer problematic messages and lectures on how to get better; that is, social networks tend not to understand and confirm the suicidal person's perspective on their pain and their distressing inability to solve their present dilemmas. Joiner et al.'s (2009) interpersonal approach, for instance, elevates clients' sense of belongingness and people's sense of being a burden to others as among the highest factors to address, as most clients tend to feel isolated and alienated from others in their social network. This approach addresses the overlapping spheres of client and culture in the process of change working diagram of the therapy contract (Figure 4.2).

The Alliance—The Intersection of All Three Spheres

The intersection of all three spheres of the diagram represents the *therapeutic alliance* with its related goals. The target of intervention is not to evaluate suicide risk levels and lower or prevent suicide per se. Suicidal risk will decrease as an alliance is built to address the acute perturbation that led to the crisis in a collaborative effort to decrease the level of distress, open new problem-solving avenues and skills, increase positive connections, establish goals, and build new hope. Also, as this alliance progresses, more time and distance are created from the initial agitation and intent. It is important to remember that suicidal risk tends to be sharply time intensive, gradually decreasing within the 48 to 72 hours following its greatest intensity.

The therapeutic alliance is strongly supported as one of the highest correlated factors with positive outcome across all psychotherapies (Horvath et al., 2011). Along with goal consensus and collaboration (Tryon & Winograd, 2011), researchers have found these elements to be a bedrock of successful treatment across all effective modes of psychotherapy. When combined with an agreed-upon rationale for treatment and its related interventions, these factors offer some of the best core sets of elements in psychotherapy that works (Constantino & Bernecker, 2014; Laska et al., 2014; Wampold & Imel, 2015). Furthermore, in a review of the factors contributing to hope, Snyder et al. (1999) made a compelling argument that hope is generated by the acceptance of a rationale that explains the nature of the problem, implies a path toward that goal, and enlists a client's motivation to go in that direction. All these elements are present in the four approaches to effective intervention in suicide being considered here. Along with the major reversal embodied in having therapists take a one-down stance and validate the distress and the plausibility of suicide given a client's situation, the working alliance interventions offer an impressive array of more seemingly counterintuitive options for practitioners. As discussed within the rationales of each approach, they all make sense in the context of the approach; however, they each represent reversals of what might make sense to a client or other helper caught in the vortex of suicidal distress or of trying to help that suicidal person. What follows is a partial set of interventions that reverse the typical patterns of the problem-generated system for the client and the therapist.

TIPPING POINTS: TRACKING GENERIC INTERVENTIONS SHARED ACROSS APPROACHES

As laid out in Chapter 4 of this volume, the generic interventions that fit the process of change model are as follows: attending to context, contextualizing and validating distress, offering rationales and reframing, normalizing, positioning and restraining, prescribing, and predicting. Each of these generic interventions is embedded in the main effective approaches to intervening in suicide: notably, the CAMS approach (Jobes, 2016), the interpersonal theory of suicide (Joiner et al., 2009), Chiles and Strosahl's (1995) approach to the suicidal patient, Beck's (2005) cognitive approach to the suicidal patient, and Linehan's (Linehan, 2014; Linehan et al., 2015) DBT approach to acutely and repeatedly suicidal individuals, among others. For further details, readers are referred to these resources and training manuals, which offer excellent guidelines and intervention suggestions. It is beyond the scope of this work to describe each approach in detail. However, our purpose here is to show their convergence on similar interventions from the process of change model. The hope is that identifying these similarities across treatments will help practitioners gain a simpler set of metaconstructs to guide their work as they home in on the model that fits them best.

With this in mind, we will take each of the process-based intervention categories in turn and offer samples from the aforementioned approaches that fit each.

Attending to Context

All of the approaches described pay close attention to the context of the suicidal person. They attend to why this trigger point is meaningful in the social and emotional contexts of that person's life and affirm the intensity of its distress as experienced by the client. As practitioners learn from their clients just how intense and hopeless they experience their situations and how isolated and alienated they feel from others who seem not to understand, intervenors find it easier to validate the pain and affirm how much sense suicide seems to make for their clients. Suicide begins to make sense in the context of people's lives. This also begins the process of (a) forming a frame for understanding suicide as a solution and (b) building a rationale within that frame for a collaborative new path to both affirm clients' values and achieve their goals through alternative solutions. Reduced risk thus follows as a by-product instead of the main goal of intervention.

Positioning and Restraining

Possibly the most powerful element of all of these problem-solving approaches comes under the idea of positioning. Taking a position that is the opposite of what is most helpful or what others would take as a key reversal of more typical helping attempts that have usually only fed into the vicious cycle of the suicidal situation. Practitioners thus spend less time and attention assessing risk factors, determining risk levels, using no-suicide contracts, and considering hospitalizations. Intervenors employing positioning with clients considering suicide would instead validate the pain, accept the prospect of suicide as a potential choice, and hold it as an option while addressing some alternate new skills and directions for the problems leading to this tipping point. This is the ultimate second-order change, or counterintuitive reversal on the part of practitioners, compared with trying to directly invalidate suicide as a choice and stop it as an option. This one-down alternate position counters both the client's solution-generated process as well as the typical reactions of their problem-generated system of those around them who typically react by invalidating the thought of suicide and do everything they can to get in its way.

Contextualizing and Validating Distress

A hallmark of all of these approaches is to affirm the client's intense pain and distress as understandable in the context of their life. Each approach emphasizes the intense distress of the person considering suicide and builds an alliance with them by validating and empathizing with them, given their context and the way they have been experiencing and dealing with it. Pure risk management misses this by focusing on interdicting the suicide itself. Furthermore, by understanding the idea of suicide within the client's lived experience and validating the felt pain, practitioners begin building the working alliance crucial to turning the tipping point of contact toward initiating a new path toward resolution.

Offering Rationales and Reframing

As noted, all of the approaches examined here reframe potential suicide as a valid choice given the client's intense distress. Furthermore, each approach offers the client a separate rationale for how the client has come to this suicidal point, how the client's repeated failed solutions make sense yet only escalate their dilemmas, and consequently how and why alternate new paths will hold more promising ways of aligning with their values and achieving their goals.

In her DBT approach, Linehan proposed that clients who chronically consider suicide often have a history of invalidation by their family and friendship networks (Linehan, 2014; Linehan et al., 2015). Thus, the threat of suicide helps draw others back to them for rescue. Thus, her interventions aim at providing radical validation, increasing distress tolerance, and teaching interpersonal effectiveness, while discouraging practitioners from reacting with distress to any ongoing suicidal gestures. Within the DBT rationales, practitioners reverse the pattern of clients experiencing invalidation, while also reversing former patterns in which clients' suicidal gestures draw others in for the relational affirmations that clients' feel they have lost or will lose. Such basic pattern reversals are at the core of the DBT approach to chronic suicidality.

Michel and Jobes's interpersonal approach stressed that suicidal people are struggling with three interpersonal factors in their social context (Jobes, 2016; Michel & Jobes, 2011). These factors include failed belongingness or having few attachments of value; perceived burdensomeness to others, seeing themselves as flawed and beyond repair; and eventual acquired suicidal capability as they gradually habituate and decrease their fear of the potential fear and pain of death. Thus, Michel and Jobes's interpersonal approach stresses a close collaborative relationship with helping others as new people skills and revised appraisals of worth evolve and put distance between intense thoughts of suicide. As practitioners operate within this frame to understand the interpersonal needs and distress of their clients, they help their clients feel affirmed and understood. This rationale then sets up the working alliance to reengage clients in their lives with others and thus move away from the intense sense of alienation and burdensomeness that was driving their thoughts of suicide. Suicidal risk once more decreases as a by-product of new problem-solving paths based on a collaborative new understanding and rationale for resolution.

Chiles and Strosahl (1995) offered a systemic and problem-solving rationale stressing that people considering suicide are confronting situations that they experience as interminable, inescapable, and intolerable (the three I's). Given that suicide behavior is an attempt to solve problems, treatment focuses on building new problem-solving skills, increasing distress tolerance, and building collaborative relationship skills with the therapist as well as socially. Practitioners affirm their clients' distress as understandable given their lived experience and validate that suicide might be an understandable choice—and one the clients might still choose if alternate solutions through the therapy contract do not pan out. Again, this rationale frames suicide as a reasonable option and then sets up a contract for the client and their intervenor to build new paths and options to affirm their values and achieve their goals.

The cognitive behavior therapy (CBT) approach matches much of these other approaches in offering the rationale that the client considering suicide has learned ineffective behaviors around distress tolerance and interpersonal relationships. Thus, practitioners work with their clients to shift clients' automatic thoughts and core beliefs about themselves and their situations, build new skills that are reinforced in treatment and socially, and decrease reinforcement for suicidal behavior. Practitioners also teach clients new skills such as mindfulness to extinguish emotional distress in the face of formerly distressing situations, in line with such rationales and instruction in mindfulness-based cognitive behavior therapy (MBCBT; Segal et al., 2002).

It may now be more apparent that these different rationales often converge on similar interventions and goals. Recall our earlier definition of hope as put forward by Snyder et al. (1999): that practitioners generate hope in clients by offering an accepted rationale that explains the problem at hand, which implies a direction to go and actions to take for resolution, and martials client motivation, whatever it may be, to go that way. Each of the four approaches described here offers such rationales, skills, and directions for clients. If the rationale and approach fit well enough with both client and practitioner and practitioners engage around these therapeutic contracts genuinely, they will most often generate the kind of hope that will eventually displace suicidal behavior.

Normalizing

It may now go without saying that all four approaches described here normalize suicidal behavior as a problem-solving choice, given the person's experience of their circumstances and life as lived. Once more, this is rather the opposite of seeing suicide as a product of some personal pathology in the patient and some implicit or explicitly abnormal or stigmatized action to be diagnosed and eliminated or "cured."

Prescribing

The notion of prescribing when it comes to suicidal behavior may initially seem paradoxical and even dangerous. How might a practitioner even consider prescribing suicidal thoughts or behavior? However, all four of these approaches do just that in an ultimate helper pattern reversal. All approaches prescribe that the suicidal client purposely reengage at some points in experiencing what brought them originally to consider suicide, or to keep logs and ratings of their suicidal thoughts and intensions.

A prime example of such *symptom prescriptions* comes from Linehan's DBT approach, in which clients are taught mindful meditation skills and then repeatedly engaged in distressing thoughts and situations as part of the approach's distress tolerance training (Linehan, 2014; Linehan et al., 2015). The goal is to directly decrease the intensity of clients' pain responses to common suicidal triggers. In a group format, this alternates with training in interpersonal effectiveness.

Similarly, in contrast with standard CBT, clients are not taught to alter the content of their thoughts in MBCBT (Segal et al., 2002); instead, clients are directed to bring their suicidal thoughts to mind and observe them merely as thoughts and related emotions. These thoughts are not then taken as literal facts or self-indictments but merely passing thoughts, as are related emotions that do not define the person or require action.

In their problem-solving approach, Chiles and Strosahl (1995) also encouraged suicidal patients to do self-monitoring tasks as homework, collecting information on their thoughts, feelings, and behavior. Clients are encouraged to attend to their daily suicidal thoughts through a log where they rate the intensity and urgency to act of each instance. Doing so inserts some distanced perspective on suicidal impulses and thoughts, along with a sense of more deliberate control and realizations that such experiences fluctuate in intensity as they come and go. Combined with a daily positive events diary completed at the end of the day, clients are encouraged to notice the balance in their lives.

From an interpersonal theory approach to suicide, Jobes (2016) stated the goal for suicidal clients as follows:

> Learning to endure the pain that results from perceptions of disconnection and burdensomeness until those perceptions can be changed—that is tranquility. Persisting in the hard work of changing distorted perceptions while refraining from impulsive responses—that is an achievement indeed. (p. 143; see also Michel & Jobes, 2011)

In their protocol, they described a prescriptive intervention that directly reengages clients considering suicide with their suicidal triggers. Similar to the chain analysis used in DBT and CBT, clients are asked to describe a discrete interpersonal event in which they intensely felt thwarted belonging or perceived burdensomeness (or both), the intensity of their experiences in the situation, and their detailed behavior. Clients then are asked to contrast the achieved outcome with their desired outcome. After this intense elicitation phase, the client and the therapist then move on to work on practical remediation. Once again, this approach directly exposes clients to the intensity of their suicidal triggers while objectifying those triggers and offering distance, perspective, and control. This is another prime example of prescribing in suicide interventions.

When seen this way, each of these seemingly paradoxical prescriptions within each of these different suicide intervention approaches make perfect sense within their respective rationales. Their joint goal is to interdict the intensity and impulsivity of the client's downward spiral while opening the threat-rigidity cycle to new perspectives and alternative directions.

Predicting

Predicting is the final overarching intervention of the four effective approaches to suicide coinciding with the tactics of a process of change approach noted earlier. Most approaches use predicting to anticipate reactions and objections to moving toward intense triggers and emotions in order to diffuse them and engage the client in collaboration. However, predicting is most often a part of anticipating potential future waves of suicidal thoughts and intentions. As opposed to the implicit goal of risk management approaches that look to eliminate suicidality, most current approaches view suicidal cycles as ongoing processes in most client's future. Practitioners often cast these cycles of distress as a "life is a roller coaster" metaphor to counter more rigid all-or-nothing thinking in which the next incident of feeling down or rejected or similar triggers are seen as relapses and cause for the next round of oscillating cycles of suicidality. Chiles and Strosahl (1995) discussed this as a means for clients to make way for future emotional suffering to minimize its impact and see it as an opportunity to look for other solutions than suicide. Across approaches, clients are often encouraged to imagine future hurdles and then list the range of new alternatives they have learned. As with DBT, they see the concepts of reconciling opposites as crucial to effective work with suicidal clients. This is the idea of finding a balance between feeling intense pain and taking action to live. Following the same rationale as a DBT position, Chiles and Strosahl (1995) said,

> The goal of establishing balance through reconciliation is essential not only for the immediate suicidal crisis, but also for developing a more robust adaptation to subsequent periods of pain and suffering . . . in the reconciling mode, these are concepts of life and death resonating against one another. (p. 77)

Clearly, all these predicting interventions serve not only to prevent relapse but also to interdict tipping points for the next vicious cycle of suicidality.

In summary, the four interventions described, along with others, converge on the process of reversing the vicious cycle of solution-generated suicidal problems within the problem-generated systems of all those who have been involved with the person who is suicidal. It remains for the practitioner to know these themes that unite approaches, adapt them to themself, and then fit them to each new client to help them use the tipping point of a suicidal situation and turn it toward a path to a life fitting their values and goals. To that end, next we will revisit a suicidal case from Chapter 4 and follow how the process of change model was used to intervene in this crisis.

APPLYING THE PROCESS OF CHANGE MODEL TO A SUICIDAL CASE

Recall the case of John from Chapter 4.[1] Briefly, John was a 28-year-old White Appalachian man. He had been in a previous marriage that ended in divorce. He then, in his words, lost a paternity case and had to help pay for a child fathered with another woman. John had worked in a local factory but had lost his job through downsizing and layoffs. The same thing happened with his most recent job working as a security guard for armored car bank deliveries. John and his current wife met on the unemployment line. They commiserated over their past marriages and ended up getting along so well they rather quickly decided to marry. At the resort town where they went on their honeymoon, John's bride began to get cold feet and thought they had rushed into things too fast. This was the final blow for John, as he then contemplated killing himself. They returned to separate apartments. John repeatedly called his wife and begged her to return and reconsider, but she continued to put him down and push him away. The night before he met with the practitioner, he had been drinking heavily, considered crashing his car into a wall on the way back from a store, and got out his loaded gun and continued drinking as he tried to work up the courage to shoot himself in the head. His family interrupted him with calls telling him how much he had to live for and continually put down the woman he had married. They recommended he call a telephone hotline. He did, and the crisis worker set an appointment for him to meet the practitioner first thing the next morning. John had evidently fallen asleep with his pistol in his lap.

Establishing a Relationship With John

By risk management profiles alone, John's profile put him in a high-risk category. He was a White middle-aged man who had experienced a sequence of

---

[1]All case examples are based on real clients, whose identities have been disguised to maintain confidentiality.

recent losses. He had been drinking heavily. Finally, he had considered several lethal plans for killing himself by driving his car into a wall or shooting himself with the handgun from his time as an armed guard—he thus had the means and ability to carry those plans out. He was also growing isolated and alienated from those he loved. The immediate tendency for most practitioners was to be drawn into the risk management mode (the *suicide attractor*, in chaos theory terms) and move quickly toward hospitalization. However, from a process-based perspective, the therapist took a very different course.

Upon hearing John's story, the therapist strongly affirmed John's pain at losing his bride, acknowledging that he had good reason for thinking of killing himself because all of his efforts to do so had failed. John said that it was a relief to have his pain and plans for killing himself validated by the practitioner because everyone, including his bride, seemed not to know how much she meant to him, how he needed her back, and how empty his life would be without her. They agreed to see how John might find a way to reopen a door to their relationship. This aligned with the first step in all effective treatment approaches, which converge on beginning a collaborative relationship to reduce suicidal risks by aligning with clients' values and goals to find a new path to achieve those goals.

Gathering Information on the Problem and Solution Patterns Surrounding It

Because the details of this case were presented in Chapter 4, only the salient points that relate its intervention to the major effective approaches described earlier will be highlighted here. First, John was particularly sensitive to another loss, given his recent pattern of significant relationship and employment losses. The potential loss of his bride thus became an acute painful trigger for him. Next, counter to his values of being more deliberate and planful, John had impulsively leapt into marrying a woman whom herself, upon reflection, doubted they had made a good choice. In the face of the high stakes of another loss, John dove into a clinging campaign with his bride, trying to convince her not to leave the new marriage. And, in the face of repeated failure, he redoubled his efforts. Upon reflection, John's goal was to reestablish his relationship with the woman he loved, and to do it in an authentic and potentially more respectful and effective way. His impulsive thoughts and plans to end his pain through suicide were also understandable, and yet ultimately ran counter to his typical more planful approach. John's family's understandable input that nothing was worth dying for, and certainly not this woman whom he had known for only a short time, had both denied his pain and distanced him from them through their efforts to help.

Coming to a Consensus on Goals, a Rationale Explaining the Problem, and Related Plans for Resolution

In line with this analysis of the vicious cycles surrounding John's dilemma, the therapist aligned with John on the goal of reestablishing his relationship with the woman he had just married. They agreed that he was a conservative and planful kind of person, and his plan going forward needed to match who he was. Suicide was certainly a choice, yet it was a final solution that needed to be considered carefully and its potential impact on all who would be affected by the suicide must be taken into consideration. John and his therapist reflected, similar to how organizations like the historical "Hemlock Society" (cf. Lester, 2013) and others advocated that individuals had a personal right to consider and plan for their own death but should do so with deliberation and with the impact and needs of all involved in mind. Furthermore, if John's current problem-solving efforts were not successful, he could always fall back on reconsidering suicide. John also agreed with the idea that forcing something, even if it might be something like ice cream on a child who was not sure if they wanted it at the time, was likely to create pushback. Arguing for their relationship with his bride was likely to meet with similar pushback, as he had found already. Furthermore, if John wanted to recapture the closeness with the woman he married, he needed to support her feelings and doubts, even if she was doubting their impulsive marriage. Telling her he understood and giving her space to miss him while she considered the future of their relationship were agreed upon as the rationale for John to back off his repeated calls, and even to make himself less available to her in the short run. John also agreed to allow the practitioner to reach out to his family, with the goal of helping them understand his pain, support giving him time to consider his future paths by holding his guns, and inviting him to stay with them while he sorted out his feelings and future choices. All these plans and related rationales were in line with John's goals and values. These also matched the consensus of all the effective approaches to suicide intervention reviewed earlier.

Break to Distance

This case was done in the context of an intervention team who operated within the process of change model. As such, there was always a staff member available to discuss all cases at a midpoint break, giving the therapist time to reflect on the case, brainstorm with a colleague, and then return to the client with a sense of support and reassurance on the potential planned intervention. This break also helps with any potential stress felt by the practitioner and counteracts their temptation to get drawn into the risk management cycles that suicidal cases like this present. This is more unique to the process of change model, yet it helps offer a supportive base for all practitioners as they more frequently engage with crises in their chosen practice approach. As we will see in Chapter 10, building in debriefing during and following regular interventions in crises is part of the generally recommended process to combat compassion fatigue or burnout (cf. Figley, 2013; Figley & Figley, 2017).

Active Problem Solving and Interventions

Once again, in summary of the interventions showing parallels with the major suicide intervention approaches reviewed earlier, each of the problem-solving plans, in line with their agreed-upon rationales, was implemented in the first session and in follow-up. John's family was contacted from the session. They were convinced of John's pain and distress and asked to support him in it; they agreed to secure his guns and ammunition and keep them in a locked place, and they agreed to have John stay with his close cousin. John agreed to call his new wife and tell her he had sought help and understood now that she needed space. He agreed not to call her until she reached out to him, and even then, he would caution them both on moving too fast back into their marriage. John then agreed to follow up with the therapist within several days and to remain in contact between now and then. All these plans and actions are well in line with the active problem-solving positions of all the effective models reviewed earlier.

Summary and Follow-Up Plans

All rationales and plans were always reviewed at the end of the first session and of all sessions that followed. As described earlier in Chapter 4, John and his family followed through with all these plans with the support of the therapist. John felt well supported and connected with the practitioner and his family, who now acknowledged his pain and supported his stance to back off his attempts to convince his new wife to return. To everyone's surprise, his wife agreed to come into counseling as a couple, where she and John agreed that their impulsive rush into marriage had spoiled a wonderful relationship. They agreed to annul the marriage and return to dating and hanging out with one another as they had before. As a result of this intervention plan and its results, John's suicide risk was reduced to nearly nothing over the process of roughly 4–6 weeks (most likely the time they would have remained on waiting lists elsewhere). He, his now former wife, and his family were grateful for the practitioner's help. This entire process again paralleled that of each of the models reviewed earlier, and it was achieved through the flexible process of change model, which we will follow through the rest of the successive chapters.

FOLLOWING THE PROCESS

In summary of the key points of this chapter, we will once more trace the points made regarding suicide and effective suicide intervention, as follows:

- When people consider suicide, practitioners need to remember that suicide is not a "thing in itself," but instead a reaction to a painful situation that is experienced as inescapable, interminable, and intolerable.

- All involved typically are drawn into what has been described as a suicide attractor, or a vortex that draws those around a potential suicide into positions of managing risks in attempts to stop the suicide. This vortex also includes practitioners if they are not careful to resist the same temptation.

- As a low base-rate event, there is no real way to predict suicide, despite the long lists of risk factors available.

- Suicide is typically triggered by one painful event that culminates in a series of stressors and creates a tipping point, like in the models of chaos and catastrophe theories explained in Part I.

- Often, direct attempts to stop suicide only exacerbate the factors contributing to it and make it worse. So-called no-suicide contracts have no support for their effectiveness. Alternative problem-solving therapy contracts are used across all effective approaches.

- Practitioners need to engage in treatment-oriented assessment instead of risk-oriented assessments.

- As we followed the process of change working diagram of the therapy contract (first discussed in Chapter 4), we found converging agreements among the four major suicide intervention models examined here.

  - In the therapist sphere, the four approaches advocate an explicitly empathetic collaborative relationship.

  - In the client sphere, the four approaches view these clients as responding to an important distressing problem serving as a trigger point that tips them toward suicide. They all acknowledge the downward spiral of growing tunnel vision views of life as well as black-and-white, all-or-none thinking and growing desperation through the threat-rigidity cycle. In addition, they all emphasize the idea of slowing down decision-making, contracting to evaluate alternatives, and increasing tolerance for distress.

– In the cultural sphere, the four approaches consider culture by addressing the nature of the culture's religious beliefs about suicide, governmental prohibitions against suicide, and sanctions following completion for survivors. They consider the nature of gender rules as well as definitions of appropriate and desirable roles and behavior. They also address how language, context, and culture channel both generic and specific solution patterns around suicide into vicious cycles of solution-generated patterns within problem-generated systems.

– Finally, turning to the alliance—or the intersection of all three spheres—all of the effective approaches discussed support an active working alliance focused on rationales and goals that fit with those of clients. Agreed-upon rationales will then help clients make sense of the new and potentially counterintuitive solution reversals that will support achieving their goals.

• Generic interventions shared across all approaches include the following:
  – attending to context,
  – positioning and offering constraints,
  – contextualizing and validating distress,
  – offering rationales and reframing,
  – normalizing,
  – prescribing, and
  – predicting.

• All of the effective approaches reviewed converge on the process of reversing the vicious cycle of solution-generated suicidal problems within the problem-generated systems of all those who have been involved with the suicidal person. The process of change model includes at a broader level all the aspects of each of the effective models reviewed in this chapter. We will find this over and again as we turn to each successive crisis, as we will see for grief and mourning in the next chapter.

7

GRIEF AND MOURNING

We will all die. This is one of life's certainties. Yet how and when death will come is uncertain. Furthermore, how we treat our own eventual death, as well as how we grieve and mourn the death of others, varies so widely that it is hard to fully grasp. Our culture, traditions, and religions guide us in our potential understandings and prescribed rituals around death. Of all crises, grief and mourning is one of the most dependent on context in our now familiar three-circle working diagram of the process of change model (Figure 4.2), consisting of spheres for the cultural context, client variables, and therapist variables. If there is one other constant that we as practitioners can rely on, however, it is that evolving vicious cycles that often emerge around death are our major target for intervention. Otherwise, our roles revolve around supporting others as they move through this inevitable transition in life for themselves and others.[1]

---

[1]Many ideas and references in this chapter relate to an unpublished dissertation I chaired in 1998, by Gerald J. Post, Jr., titled, *A Personal-Contextual Model of Bereavement*, in partial fulfillment of the requirements for the degree of Doctor of Psychology, in the School of Professional Psychology of the Wright State University.

https://doi.org/10.1037/0000445-008
Crisis Intervention: Using Tipping Points to Achieve Transformative Change in Therapy, by J. S. Fraser

Again, there has been so much written about death and dying, the nature and circumstances of loss, and the varieties of responses to death that a complete treatment of the topic falls far beyond the scope of this chapter. Instead, we will focus first on what has not been useful and then on how the process of change view fits with some of the most promising approaches to treatment.

As is our custom in this book, we will first present some case examples that we will return to at the end of this chapter. Following these initial cases, we will review the history of perspectives on grief, including phase and stage models, and discuss how they fail to capture grief and mourning across spectrums and how they have often exacerbated the problems they seek to resolve. We will explore the following questions:

- What is grief?
- How can it be viewed as normal?
- Do grieving and mourning even need intervention, and if so, how and when?
- When might solutions become the problem on the part of individuals, helpful others, and practitioners?

Finally, we will explore promising approaches to grieving as a normal process, to fitting needed interventions to the style of grieving, and to applying an adaptive grieving model. These models will then be illustrated by revisiting the initial cases, as viewed through the process of change perspective.

First, consider the case of Hope[2] and her family. Hope was a 22-year-old White Appalachian woman who came to the practitioner's office with her 5-year-old son. She had been having trouble eating and sleeping, and she had also been experiencing a range of strange and frightening things. Furthermore, her son was getting out of control, and she needed help with him. Initially, her son was so disruptive in the office that the therapist asked another staff person to watch him in another area.

Hope then shared she had recently felt that someone was outside her bedroom door at night, but when she checked, no one was there. Several nights, she awakened and saw a person standing next to a casket in her bedroom. Most recently, as she stared at herself in the mirror, she could see her face melting.

When the therapist asked what had happened recently in her life, Hope told of a very close cousin who was run out of town by her dominant mother, who was essentially the matriarch of her extended Appalachian family. Shortly thereafter, her cousin was decapitated in a car accident in Tennessee

---

[2]All case examples are based on real clients, whose identities have been disguised to maintain confidentiality.

as his car slid under a truck in a rainstorm. The entire family was very upset and angry. At the funeral, they had an open casket, as was their Appalachian family tradition, wherein the undertakers had attempted to recreate their cousin's features in wax. Since the funeral, Hope had some contact with several sisters who were also distressed but uncertain what to do. Hope's main support was her boyfriend, who appeared to be involved with some activity that required him to be frequently out of town and also to carry a gun. She had been late to work because of oversleeping, and she often needed to take off work to handle her son. She wanted to know how the therapist could help.

Now consider the case of Mr. C. Mr. C was a 75-year-old recently widowed Korean man who was brought to treatment by his son. Mr. C had a history of hospitalization and outpatient treatment over the past 20 years due to recurrent episodes of schizophrenia, paranoid type. He had responded well to psychotropic medication and counseling over the years and had remained compliant with this treatment. His last hospitalization was 5 years ago, following the death of his daughter in a car accident. His son reported that since the death of his wife 3 months ago, Mr. C had been somewhat withdrawn, tearful, and confused, with possible memory loss (e.g., problems remembering names and appointments). Mr. C also had recurrent thoughts of death and had declining adaptive functioning (e.g., he had not maintained a regular diet, bathed irregularly, and neglected household chores).

Upon interview, Mr. C presented with adequate personal hygiene and was dressed appropriately. He was well oriented to person, place, and time. His speech was well organized and appropriate. There were no overt indications of disorganized thought, looseness of associations, tangential thought, or pressured speech. He did, however, report hearing his wife's voice in the evening and early morning, reassuring him that she is okay and in the presence of Jesus. He denied suicidal ideation. He acknowledged some minor difficulties with taking care of himself since his wife's death as well as remembering day-to-day events, places where he had put items, and the names of recently introduced people. His mood appeared moderately depressed; his affect appeared flat, although some range in emotional expressiveness was demonstrated (e.g., irritability with his son and some others). His son feared another psychotic break and hospitalization.

Finally, consider my experience some years ago, when I had the privilege of serving as a Semester at Sea professor teaching undergraduate students from across the United States and other countries. We sailed halfway around the world over a 4-month semester, stopping at ports in different countries and adjusting our curriculum and syllabi to each country and culture. One of the three courses I taught was Death and Dying. I was amazed, as were the students, by the wide range of perspectives on death and rituals around death encountered from culture to culture.

Ghana was perhaps one of the more interesting countries in how they celebrate deaths. Large community gatherings are valued; the more people who attend, the greater honor for the deceased. In the city of Accra, we saw large billboards throughout the city advertising the passing of an honored family member and inviting all to attend the celebration. Those with more resources often order what might be called a "vanity casket" that depicts the focus of the person's life. We visited a casket factory, where we saw a tribal chief's casket that replicated his throne, another was in the shape of a shoe for a shoemaker, and there was a lovely fish for a fisherman; the most unique for us was one replicating a Coke machine. For people dying younger than age 50 or 60 years, black and red robes were common; for elders, the colors were black and white. Bands led parades down streets in villages to large feasts. Yet, reflecting again on vicious cycles, the government was encouraging less elaborate and expensive celebrations, as many families were left destitute following these funerals.

Yet maybe one of the most surprising traditions in Ghana surrounded the death of children—typically viewed as a tragedy in most Western cultures. A lecturer at the University of Ghana (personal communication, October 1, 2018) told us that children are not named immediately after birth in case they died early in their life. In the case of such early death before naming, the child was revered as an angel recalled by the gods and thus celebrated for that. A similar pattern was seen earlier in parts of Brazil: in certain cultures, the death of some children was seen as a cause for great joy or else a matter of indifference (Scheper-Hughes, 1992). In some instances, such as in the death of very young children, they may be seen as becoming *Valerio de Anjinhos* (angel babies) descending directly to heaven without having to suffer the burdens of life and loss of innocence. At other times, a child or infant's death may be experienced as a relief of the burden of raising another child in a life of hunger, violence, and poverty. Context and beliefs are everything.

When we stopped in Vietnam, we found that the Vietnamese people also celebrated the death of loved ones with *Dam Gio* or death day. The traditional period of formal mourning is often 2 years, after which other life changes may be planned, with varying intervals of celebrations of the death in the first year and then spanned out over the next. Yet the anniversary of a loved one's death is celebrated yearly on that day from then onward.

Sadly, the entire ship joined in a funeral ceremony upon the untimely death of the husband of one of the administrators. The couple's children sailed with us all and became well known and loved by the students and faculty alike. To honor that passing, the captain ordered enough white roses for all students, faculty, and crew; and each tossed their rose one at a time off the stern of the ship, reflecting on death in their own way as the captain sailed the ship in a broad circle and the ship's crew sang hymns. This was both touching and unique, as are most all varying rituals across cultures, times, and places. Context and meaning are everything.

Stroebe et al. (1993) defined three terms associated with loss as follows: "*bereavement* refers to the objective situation of having lost someone significant; *grief* is the emotional response to one's loss; and *mourning* denotes the actions and manner of expressing grief, which often reflect the mourning practices of one's culture" (p. 5, emphasis in original). Each of the cases just described marked significant losses. Each involved the response of significant others in a cultural context, and all mourned in their own unique ways. Yet how might a practitioner respond to such widely different cases, contexts, and practices? Is there some significant integration of theory and practice that might guide a practitioner on how to intervene or not in each instance? We explore these topics next.

A HISTORY OF GRIEF MODELS

Relating back to our initial discussion in Chapter 1 of the origins of formal crisis intervention, we revisit the work of Erich Lindemann (1944) following the Cocoanut Grove fire in Boston, Massachusetts. His focus was on the reactions of survivors of that disaster to their loss. In his classic work on the symptomology and management of acute grief, Lindemann found a remarkable consistency among 101 survivors. He described a syndrome, which he termed *acute grief*, immediately after a crisis, which may also be delayed, exaggerated, or apparently absent. He went on to describe what he called *normal grief*, which showed a remarkable consistency of sighing, preoccupation with images of the deceased, guilt, hostility, and disrupted daily living. Because most people seemed to avoid the intense emotions and experiences of grieving, his interventions (termed *grief work*, which was coined by Freud in 1917) focused on having survivors remain with the intensity of the experiences until they became emancipated and able to form new relationships—or a clear pattern reversal. This reflected the Freudian psychodynamic tradition of grief work in which Lindemann was trained. Lindemann (1944) went on, however, to chronicle what he termed as *morbid grief reactions*, or distortions of what he found to be normal grief, including *delayed grief* in the face of pressing tasks. He also described *distorted reactions*, which included overactivity without a sense of loss, acquiring symptoms of the lost loved one, psychosomatic symptoms, hostility toward others, reactions resembling psychotic behaviors, lasting losses of social interaction, self-harming, and agitated depression. Given the nearly uniform wish to master the grief through avoidance, the essence of Lindemann's early prescription for the practitioner was sharing the patient's grief work, through accepting the pain of the loss, turning toward it, and working through it in line with the prevailing psychodynamic perspective of the day. The tradition was clearly to support the counterintuitive pattern reversal of repeated denial, thus interdicting the vicious cycle and initiating a new tipping point for a more positive virtuous cycle. Much of this tradition continues.

Although many of these normative observations have been roundly criticized and revised, they set the groundwork for studying grief, intervening in crises of loss, and laying out general paths for intervention. Many of these themes persist today, including a search for what is "normal" grief, the nature of complex or complicated grief, traumatic grief reactions, prolonged grief, age-related reactions (e.g., in childhood, adolescence, or in aging), and specific reactions to the type of relationships lost. The other major theme has been to plot and discover the so-called uniform phases and stages of grief. We turn next to these.

Stage, Phase, and Task Models

In many ways, the bereavement literature has some of its roots in Freud's early views on attachment, put forward in his work, *Mourning and Melancholia* (Freud, 1922). These models view grief as an emotional process triggered by loss and have been referred to as *depression models of grief*. Going forward and based on the work on attachment by John Bowlby (1969, 2005), many authors based their work on themes of attachment, loss, separation, and recovery. Currently, the predominant paradigms in grief counseling and therapy have retained the psychodynamic concepts of bonding, separation, letting go, and reinvesting in new relationships.

This paradigm forms the basis for many *stage models of grief*. The most influential of these models is Elisabeth Kübler-Ross's (1969) stage theory of dying, described in her seminal book, *On Death and Dying*. Based on her work with patients with cancer confronting their own potential deaths, Kübler-Ross's five-stage model of denial, anger, bargaining, depression, and acceptance has become so popular in both professional and social arenas that the stages might be recited by students, practitioners, politicians, comedians, and a wide range of others. The stages metaphor has caught on given its simple framework for normalizing grief and offering guidelines for its resolution.

Several similar stage models have been synthesized into three main phases, the first of which is characterized by shock, numbness, disbelief, denial, or disorganization. In the middle phase, or working phase, the mourner, experiencing intense affect and distress, comes to terms with the loss and resulting changes. The final phase involves resolution, reconciliation, relief, or reconstruction.

The widespread application of stage models has led to modified models referred to as *task models* (Worden, 2018; Worden & Winokuer, 2021), which shift the role of the griever from passive observer to active participant in the process. The grief process is viewed as a series of sequential tasks or goals that must be accomplished to successfully achieve relief after loss. Worden's four tasks, for example, are first to accept the reality of the loss, next to process the pain of the loss, then to adjust to an environment where the deceased is missing, and, finally, to emotionally relocate and memorialize the dead person in a way that one can move on with life.

The stage, phase, and task metaphors have served to support increased interest in bereavement and the grief process over several decades. They have also made such sense to people that they have been taught and applied widely. Kübler-Ross's (1969) work, for example, initiated renewed interest in grief and loss, made it the focus of scientific inquiry, and prompted an examination of beliefs about grief and mourning in Western culture. To a great extent, hospice in the United States, and its benefits to dying individuals and their families, owes a great debt to her work.

However, stage, phase, and task theories tend to obscure the complexity of grief responses attributable to individual differences and contextual variables (Wortman & Silver, 1989; Wortman et al., 1993). Recall here our discussion of generic and specific variations of crisis patterns from Part I. Generic patterns may be common within a given cultural context; however, they may take on a unique "spin" by individual or specific factors or they may be entirely different within another cultural context. Although stage models are helpful in viewing grief as a process, Wortman et al. (1993) suggested that the models "cannot account for the diversity in outcomes that occur in response to loss events and cannot explain, for example, why one person is devastated by a particular loss and another emerges relatively unscathed" (p. 352). This critique is again aligned with the premises of the process view of open systems. A model that explains a human process should be universally applicable, yet stage, phase, and task models may be an artifact of modern Western culture with culturally embedded values of autonomy.

Stage, phase, and task theories have also not been well supported by empirical studies (Konigsberg, 2011) even as they remain popular in general

Western culture. As a result, the Kübler-Ross (1969) five-stage model along with many other stage, phase, and task models have been moved to the sidelines in academic and clinical practice (Friedman & James, 2009). Citing Konigsberg (2011), Neimeyer (2000), and Worden (2002), James and Gilliland (2016) offered the following list refuting many of the ideas on grief that have been associated with stage theories:

1. The common assumptions concerning "stages of grief" are not supported.

2. Placing time limitations on grief is inappropriate.

3. The withholding or suppression of sadness in response to bereavement is not necessarily pathological.

4. Insistence on severing ties or detaching oneself from lost objects denies lifelong bonding and usefulness of positive memories.

5. One-size-fits-all models do not work because each individual griever's experience is unique. Grief is not a unitary phenomenon but rather a multidimensional, interactive, individual experience for every bereaved person, based on a complex set of interwoven variables.

6. There are no fixed beginning and ending points in grieving.

7. While grief does not end, it does change. (p. 421)

All of these points are directly aligned with the process of change perspective. Yet in the face of these critiques, where might we go from here? Stage models, like the one first advanced by Kubler-Ross in 1969, are widely criticized as inadequate and simplistic. However, they have been emulated, along with phase and task models, by many others and are relied on heavily by health care professionals and others when responding to grief reactions. These models are linear and parsimonious, easy to understand and communicate with others, and readily lend themselves to applications across situations. Appealing ideas can take on lives of their own, even in the absence of empirical or other scientific support, especially when a more compelling explanation has not yet been developed.

Furthermore, attempting to force a Western cultural template on those from other cultures and subcultures has often resulted in at best neutral results, but oftentimes has exacerbated the very problems they set out to resolve. This echoes what we discussed in Chapter 4 about Western-trained practitioners' attempts to help residents of Sri Lanka following the devastating tsunami by teaching their culturally based ideas of posttraumatic stress disorder, which resulted in problematic ends. Wolfelt (2007) argued that goals such as treating grief as a syndrome, promoting client disengagement from the deceased and terminating the relationship, having the client finish a series of tasks, using a recovery or resolution model to return to a preloss state, and considering grief as a crisis where balance can be reachieved, among other targets, can cause more harm than good. This reflects the essence of Part I of this book: the basic, and mistaken, premise of crisis intervention has been the implicit goal of returning systems in crisis to their homeostatic balance, or their precrisis state.

In the face of these critiques, where might we go from here? Based on the limitations of existing models, a consensus has emerged in the literature that there is a need for models that are more flexible, accommodate more variability in coping responses, are less prescriptive, account for contextual variables, and respect individual differences (Gergen, 2022; Kastenbaum & Thuell, 1995; Stroebe et al., 1992). As we will see, this prescription turns out to be a close fit to the process of change perspective at the heart of this book. This also leads to questions such as whether grief intervention is helpful or even needed, and if so, when, for whom, and what are the best approaches to intervention.

INTERVENING IN GRIEF AND MOURNING

Given this quest for more flexible approaches to grief counseling, where does this leave the practitioner regarding intervention? In many ways, most practitioners have been trained in the general application of the now more dated and problematic stage, phase, and task models. Furthermore, there has been a lively debate on whether general grief counseling even works.

The Debate Over What Works

Currier, Neimeyer, and colleagues reviewed more than 60 controlled studies of grief intervention that included a control group in some form and came to several conclusions and recommendations (Currier et al., 2008; Neimeyer & Currier, 2009). They concluded, "Consistent with the majority of smaller-scale reviews, our tests of overall effectiveness failed to yield an overly encouraging picture of grief therapies. . . . Of the overall analyses, grief therapies did outperform no-intervention control conditions immediately following the intervention" (Neimeyer & Currier, 2009, p. 4). However, follow-up an average of 8 months later failed to find intervention effects at all, in contrast to general psychotherapy across all problems using bona fide treatments, which typically show large effects at the end of treatment and show enduring improvement (Wampold & Imel, 2015). So, what does this mean for intervening in grief? Should it not be done? Neimeyer and Currier (2009) went on to say that "beyond this general conclusion, other analyses revealed that some treatments showed little benefit or even negative effects, whereas other therapies enjoyed impressive effectiveness" (p. 4). Whereas universal interventions showed little benefits compared to simply the passage of time, more focused, planned interventions in incidents referred to as *complicated grief* tended to show impressive success.

Much of the research on grief counseling effectiveness converges on the finding that it is, in fact, quite useful for individuals who are contending with substantial clinical distress, such as complicated or complex grief reactions. This finding is quite relevant to events occurring globally at the time of this writing, with recent massive numbers of complicated and traumatic deaths associated with the Russian invasion of Ukraine and with the conflict between Israel and Hamas in Gaza and the West Bank.

In the face of these findings of little effect for grief interventions in general, Stroebe et al. (2005) said,

> Nevertheless, there are bereaved individuals who need help and who derive benefits from grief counseling and therapy. Most typically, these are individuals who have been unable to cope with their loss and for whom the grief reaction has in some way "gone wrong." The term complicated grief is used. (p. 410)

In their meta-analysis of the prevention and treatment of complicated grief, Wittouck et al. (2011) concluded, "Treatment interventions can effectively diminish complicated grief symptoms. Preventive interventions, on the other hand, do not appear to be effective" (p. 69). Upon reviewing the grief intervention literature, Bonanno and Lilienfeld (2008) concluded the following:

> [M]ost bereaved people do not need and will not benefit from clinical intervention. Moreover, when treatment is focused appropriately on bereaved people who do seek or need professional help and when interventions are appropriately tailored, treatment effects will be comparable with those of other forms of psychotherapy. (p. 377)

Schut (2010) agreed:

> We know now that it is not effective to offer unsolicited help to bereaved people for no other reason than they have lost somebody. . . . With regard to full-blown therapy for complicated grief, the picture has always been more positive. Many of the well-designed controlled intervention studies for complicated grief do show modest but lasting results, just like most other psychotherapeutic interventions. (p. 9)

Complex Grief or Complicated Grief Disorder as an Intervention Target

What is meant by complicated grief? Formerly known as complicated grief disorder, *persistent complex bereavement disorder* causes sufferers to feel extreme yearning for a deceased loved one, usually over a prolonged period. Feelings of longing are often accompanied by destructive thoughts and behaviors as well as by general impairment in resuming normal life. Persistent complex bereavement disorder is included in the chapter in the *Diagnostic and Statistical Manual of Mental Disorders, Fifth Edition* (*DSM-5*), that outlines areas for further study (American Psychiatric Association, 2013).

According to the *DSM-5*, the criteria for complicated grief are broadly that the patient experienced the death of a loved one at least 6 months previously, and at least one of the following symptoms has been present longer than expected, taking into account the person's social or cultural environment:

- intense and persistent yearning for the deceased
- frequent preoccupation with the deceased
- intense feelings of emptiness or loneliness
- recurrent thoughts that life is meaningless or unfair without the deceased
- a frequent urge to join the deceased in death

In addition, at least two of the following symptoms have been recorded for at least 1 month:

- feeling shocked, stunned, or numb since a loved one's death
- feelings of disbelief or inability to accept the loss
- rumination about the circumstances or consequences of the death
- anger or bitterness about the death
- experiencing pain that the deceased suffered, or hearing or seeing the deceased
- trouble trusting or caring about others
- intense reactions to memories or reminders of the deceased
- avoidance of reminders of the deceased, or the opposite—seeking out reminders to feel close to the deceased
- the symptoms cause substantial distress for the sufferer or impact significantly on areas of functioning and cannot be attributed to other causes

The New Wave of Grief Interventions

Given the research just reviewed, we describe a set of recommended approaches for practitioners to consider, all of which align with the process of change model we have been following throughout these chapters linking all effective approaches across all crises. Neimeyer (2001) suggested that "a 'new wave' of grief theory is emerging that reflects a changing *zeitgeist* about the role of loss in human experience" (p. 3). Neimeyer further described this as follows:

Among the common elements of these newer models are

- skepticism about the universality of a predictable emotional trajectory that leads from psychological disequilibrium to readjustment, coupled with an appreciation of more complex patterns of adaptation;

- a shift away from the presumption that successful grieving requires withdrawal of psychic energy from the one who has died, and toward a recognition of the potentially healthy role of continued symbolic bonds with the deceased person;

- attention to broadly cognitive processes entailed in mourning, supplementing the traditional focus on the emotional consequences of loss;

- a de-emphasis on universal syndromes of grieving and a focus of "local" practices for accommodating loss among specific categories of the bereaved or various (sub)cultural groups;

- a greater awareness of the implications of major loss for the individual's sense of identity, often necessitating deep revisions in his or her self-definition;

- increased appreciation of the possibility of life-enhancing "post-traumatic growth" as one integrates the lessons of loss; and

- a broadened focus not only on the experience of individual survivors but also on the patterns and processes by which loss is negotiated in families and wider social contexts. (pp. 3–4)

THE PROCESS OF CHANGE IN GRIEF INTERVENTION

Recalling the basic concepts of the process of change perspective on crises and crisis intervention, the process of change approach offers a close fit with what the field of grief intervention has been calling for. Remember that the process view of human open systems is focused on continual change rather than homeostatic stability or return to precrisis states. Different outcomes typically evolve from similar beginnings (referred to as *multifinality* in complex systems terms), and similar outcomes may evolve from very different beginnings (referred to as *multideterminism* in complex system terminology). The context and intervening process is what helps shape eventual outcomes. The process of change view aligns with the social constructionist perspective on context (Gergen, 1985, 2022), which suggests that our worldviews and lived realities coevolve from social interactions within cultural and local language, beliefs, and traditions. It also emphasizes the influence of chance and contingency in the lives of people, such that relatively minor or even catastrophic changes tend to evolve either positively or negatively in what is often referred to as *virtuous or vicious cycles*. Change such as death may be relatively assimilated to or accommodated in the experience of some as they move forward in their lives, yet it may initiate escalating vicious cycles of distress and disruption in the lives of others. Similarly, given a *fitting shift* in such vicious cycles that may occur by chance or by design at a new tipping point with the help of a practitioner, a *more flexible* virtuous cycle may begin.

The process of change perspective also aligns with current psychotherapy literature that emphasizes the ideas of *flexibility* and *fit* (Fraser, 2018, pp. 55–57). Flexibility may be considered broadly as a positive position for both individuals confronting change and practitioners helping people in distress to negotiate that change. For example, rigid adherence to ignoring the reality of a loss or death on one hand and to consistently attending to the distress and circumstances resulting from a loss or death on the other hand typically result in escalating cycles fitting the aforementioned characteristics of complex bereavement. Resolution, in such instances, aligned with the literature, involves survivors adapting more flexibility in attending to both the distress and negativity of the loss, as well as the history or positives in the lost relationship as they engage in the realistic tasks involved in adjusting to life following the loss in a cyclical alternating way (Fraser, 1995b, 1998a, 2018; Norcross, 2002). Similarly, for practitioners, the recommended positions with those being helped are to *flex* to the apparent needs and goals of survivors, while *fitting* their interventions to the language, culture, beliefs, and context in which those people and their significant others live (Fraser, 1995b, 2001, 2018; Norcross, 2002). The process of change perspective suggests that people in their personal and social contexts most often will evolve to assimilate and accommodate to death and loss and, at best, may benefit by significant others or practitioners sharing that journey in compassionate, accepting, and affirming ways. Thus, the main target of any designed intervention to help around such significant loss is when survivors or those close to them (or both) request help in moving beyond the respective vicious cycles of what we have termed *solution-generated problems* within potentially *problem-generated systems*.

This brings us to several of the newer and more promising approaches to intervention around death, grief, and mourning, each of which fits well with the process of change approach. The first approach addresses the best positions for helpers with those moving through uncomplicated grief. The other approaches address intervening with more prolonged complex grief in a way that turns vicious repeated cycles toward newer and more positive ends. Finally, we will revisit the first two cases introduced at the beginning of the chapter.

Being There With Most Grieving People

Recall once more the concepts of solution-generated problems and problem-generated systems. Also, recalling the concept of attractors in chaos theory, a death tends to draw all around it, survivors and helping systems alike, into culturally prescribed patterns of helping with the loss. However, as we have found, when extra help is not needed, such unsolicited help can maintain the grieving process—or worse, exacerbate it—creating a solution-generated problem pattern now found in the literature. Therefore, practitioners and other related helpers are best advised to join with and allow the grief and mourning process to evolve more naturally.

In keeping with the research that shows little or no significant change or even harm from intervention in grief where there is little unusual distress and neither the aggrieved person nor others are soliciting help, Altmaier (2011) offered some guidelines for clinicians, family, and friends, termed *focusing on the relationship* and what has also been referred to as "being there." This finding is, of course, well aligned with the universally supported importance of the relationship in general psychotherapy (cf. Duncan et al., 2010; Norcross, 2002; Wampold & Imel, 2015), in which a positive relationship has consistently been found to account for 60% to 80% of the variance in change across modes of psychotherapy. Altmaier's suggestions all come under what might fit in the colloquial phrase, "If it ain't broke, don't fix it!" These guidelines include the following:

- Be an *empathic presence*, including listening, silence, and support; being nonjudgmental; and allowing feelings both positive and negative to be expressed.

- Offer *gentle conversation*, avoiding easy answers and clichés.

- *Provide available space* by helping the client find support, engaging in things that will help in the moment, and listening to what they need.

- *Elicit trust* and affirming, through shared understanding and compassion, that the survivors will be able to survive hard times, recover, and grow.

Of course, all these stances will vary and need to be adjusted to the language, culture, and relationship of the helpful others or practitioner involved. An example in my own practice was the case of Mary, who was in her late 70s and had been a client earlier, along with her husband of more than 50 years. They had originally come for help with their two adult sons who were both brilliant yet seemed to be failing to reach their potential. Following a positive therapeutic collaboration and the resolution of that issue, Mary recontacted me some years later. She had recently endured the very painful death of her beloved husband. It seemed she simply could not cry or even recall his face. After sharing her current situation, we eventually scheduled a time to meet one morning by a pond she and her husband would regularly visit in the morning and bring pastries and the newspaper. We shared some quiet time and talked gently about the wonderful relationship and great times she and her husband had shared over the years. While this might also be cast as a reversal of Mary's "remembering to forget" the pain of her loss, it was also an example of simply being there with her and the memory of her beloved husband. We touched based a time or two thereafter. Finally, some months down the road, we crossed paths again. Mary said she had moved into a retirement community that she loved and had a circle of lovely new friends. We again shared our fondness for her husband and her pride in their sons' lives.

The Dual Process Model

When clients are requesting help around more complex and complicated grief, there is a newer option that addresses both actively grieving and making meaning of the loss and beginning to move forward given the loss. This oscillating model deliberately embraces what is often a common oscillating pattern for people more naturally attempting to resolve loss. Adapting more process-based approaches to grief, Stroebe and Schut (2001a, 2001b, 2008, 2010) proposed what they called a *dual process model* (DPM) of grief. Their research on the grief process identified two overall types of coping mechanisms: The first is termed *loss oriented* (LO), and the second is *restoration oriented* (RO). Loss-oriented coping mechanisms include ruminating about the deceased, experiencing sadness and often tears, and recalling life together before the death and events related to the death. Restoration-oriented coping refers to the secondary stresses related to the bereaved addressing new tasks previously managed by the deceased, role changes, the assumption of new identities, and other practical matters needing to be addressed around the death, such as funerals, economic issues, and more. Stroebe and Schut proposed that *both* orientations are needed for survivors to adequately move through the grieving process. Problems may arise when survivors *rigidly* stick with one mode or the other and escalate through inevitable vicious cycles. Stroebe and

Schut postulated that the more adaptive process involves *oscillation* between the two as the survivor gradually adapts.

Stroebe and Schut (2016) described this process as follows:

> According to the DPM, both LO and RO are part of the grieving process; one needs to attend to each orientation in order to adjust to a world in which the loved person is no longer physically present. This brings us to a feature of the DPM which is one of its most distinctive, namely, the notion of *oscillation*. Oscillation is a dynamic, regulatory coping process, based on the principle, indicated earlier, that the bereaved person will at times (have to—in order to come to terms with the bereavement) confront aspects of loss (deal with LO stressors), while at other times he or she will (have to) avoid them. The same applies to restoration (RO) tasks: At times, these need to be attended to (at which times LO coping cannot take place) and this goes hand-in-hand with avoidance of RO at other times too. But one cannot cope the whole time, it is exhausting to do so a lot of the time; *time off* is needed, where nonbereavement-related activities are followed or when the person simply relaxes and recuperates. Life goes on, and this, in and of itself, can at times be quite beneficial and healing. The components described earlier combine to make coping with bereavement—according to the DPM—a complex regulatory process of confrontation and avoidance. (pp. 99–100)

The dual process model integrates many of the assumptions of the attachment model of Bowlby (2005) and the task model of Worden and Winokuer (2021), yet it offers a process-based model of a *flexible* grief resolution perspective that may serve well when a practitioner encounters the rigid escalating vicious cycles of more complicated grief. This model has spurred extensive interest and research to see if it models general bereavement experiences and whether interventions based on the dual process model are more effective than traditional grief interventions. Fiore (2021) consulted 20 databases for publications related to the dual process model, finding 474 articles and conducting 86 full-text reviews with 22 quantitative or mixed method studies. Fiore concluded that the dual process model "accurately represents the bereavement experience and can be used to understand how bereaved individuals cope. [And furthermore] Interventions based upon the DPM may be more effective than traditional grief therapy" (p. 414).

Although the dual process model began with a focus on individuals making meaning within their cultural context as they evolved through their loss, the model has evolved to include the same oscillating process with families and related social systems involved as well (Stroebe & Schut, 2015). A most recent step, maybe of most interest to our discussion of crises and crisis intervention, is Stroebe and Schut's (2016) incorporation of what they term *overload* in the lives of the bereaved. Intense grief, followed by the addition of the potential for overwhelming stress that may come from multiple life events occurring all at once, may create overload. (This is likely particularly relevant to those experiencing deaths of loved ones within ongoing wars noted at this writing.) Stroebe and Schut (2016) explained this by saying that overload may involve the following:

> too much to deal with on the loss-oriented side. If more than one bereavement occurs simultaneously or in quick succession, it may be difficult to grieve for the different losses at the same time. However, overload can also derive from experiencing too many restoration stressors. Interpersonal difficulties (e.g., quarrels and disagreements) may contribute to a feeling of overload. Furthermore, too many stressors may occur in both loss and restoration categories (e.g., multiple bereavements combined with financial and rehousing consequences). Finally, making it even more multifaceted—loss- or restoration-oriented overload may be augmented by an overload of things that have nothing to do with the bereavement, either directly or indirectly (e.g., extraneous to bereavement demands on one's time; too much to do at one's workplace). (pp. 101–102)

In discussing strategies for using the dual process model, Humphrey (2009) suggested that the practitioner do the following: (1) identify both the loss and its avoidance, and the restoration and confrontation responses the client currently uses; (2) identify evidence of oscillation already present; (3) explain the dual process model and normalize and validate the model as it relates to the client's current situation; (4) identify any extreme avoidance or loss-oriented behaviors; then (5) prescribe the process of oscillation to be done more deliberately by the survivor, alternating between loss-oriented days, where both sad or distressing emotions as well as positive reflections on the diseased are felt, and restoration-oriented days where tasks of life after the loss are attended to; and, finally, (6) *not* to push clients toward resolution and instead let the oscillation work. A related advantage of such prescriptions and the deliberate practice of things that formerly felt out of control is that it puts the survivor back in the "driver's seat" with their grieving process, giving them control of what formerly felt out of control. From the process of change model's set of general interventions, this is clearly a prescription.

The more recent addition to the dual process model feeds directly into what is usually termed *complex grieving*, in which an individual or social network shuts down or becomes triggered into vicious cycles around loss issues, restoration issues, or both simultaneously. A complementary realization of dual processes of grieving has also emerged from a study by Martin and Doka (2000) of broad gender differences in grieving. They originally observed that women generally were more open to expression of emotions around grief, or an affective path, or what they called *intuitive grieving*, whereas men were more often instrumental in their resolution efforts. Eventually, these authors abandoned their gender-anchored descriptions and moved toward describing grieving as a simultaneous path of *both* intuitive and instrumental engagement (Doka & Martin, 2011). Relating to more complex grieving, they now advocate an *integrative* approach that blends modalities and approaches fitting with affective strategies, behavioral strategies, cognitive strategies, and spiritual strategies. This stance aligns closely with the process-based approach, which advocates *flexing* the practitioner's approach to the survivor's worldview and *fitting* frames to help make sense of gradual shifts out of vicious cycles and toward more positive paths (see also Fraser, 1995a, 1998a, 2001, 2018, 2020).

Making Meaning of Loss and Growing Beyond

Recall once again that the process of change approach to intervention in perceived crises is closely related to social constructionism and how we all make meaning of our experienced world in a gradual, co-evolving way within our social contexts. Remember as well that the thesis of the perspective is that crises like death and loss, if taken advantage of by all involved, are often springboards to positive change.

Growing Beyond Loss

More recent research on grief intervention converges on the conclusion that the most useful target for intervention is complex or complicated grief. Particularly in the instance of violent loss, Currier et al. (2006) found that failure to find meaning in such losses is a crucial pathway to complicated grief. Neimeyer and colleagues conducted extensive work on what they term "meaning-making" as a critical element of how survivors move best through loss (Neimeyer, 2000, 2001; Neimeyer et al., 2014). Death and loss will come into everyone's life; yet even for those of us who try to remain aware of that fact, losing a loved one still tends to demand either assimilating or accommodating that loss into our views of the world as safe and stable. This is especially true in instances of sudden or violent death. Over and again, across perspectives, survivors have been found to experience the best resolutions and movement forward in their lives through the process of finding meaning in the death as it related to their life and the lives of others.

Posttraumatic Growth

This position on the potential positive resolution of loss and traumatic and complex grief is also reflected in the research around the idea of *posttraumatic growth* (Calhoun & Tedeschi, 2014a, 2014b; Tedeschi & Calhoun, 2004a, 2004b; Tedeschi et al., 2015), as discussed in Chapter 5 (this volume). The essence of this research is that once again there is a paradox or counterintuitive reversal in outcomes of traumatic events or losses when those involved engage in the events with an eye toward making new meaning and facilitating positive new paths. Reflecting on the concepts in Part I of this book, this is a prime example of second-order change and potential transformative change. Linley and Joseph reported that posttraumatic growth has been found in a wide range of crises, including cancer, the Oklahoma City bombing, sexual assault, plane crashes, and combat (Joseph et al., 2004; Linley & Joseph, 2004a, 2004b, 2005; Linley et al., 2006). Of particular relevance to grief and mourning is a study of persons who lost family members to death and were interviewed before and after the loss (Davis et al., 1998). Those who either made sense of the loss through faith or related ideas or found something positive in the experience through improved family relationships, for example, were less distressed 6 months after the death and experienced better adjustment. Crises such as death and traumatic loss, far from needing to be settled back to precrisis states, often result in *positive trajectories* in the lives of survivors. This realization that helping survivors turn toward positive recollections of the deceased and potentially positive future directions is found in the latest dual process model's directions for survivors to *deliberately* spend equal time in sad reflections as well as positive reflections of life with the lost loved one. More recent research has supported this balance as more helpful than pure immersion in clearly sad and distressing emotions alone.

Thus, practitioners are advised to be cautious of being drawn into the vortex of regularly offering grief interventions in the majority of instances. Most people move through the grieving process reasonably well without professional intervention. However, when survivors or members of their social networks seek help and when telltale rigidity and vicious cycles become apparent, a sensitive application of a variation of the dual process model can help all involved make more meaning of the loss and shift their vicious cycles of solution-generated problems and problem-generated systems while also moving forward with making a new life in the face of the loss. This holds the best promise of moving all toward more satisfying growth in their lives as they move forward.

APPLYING THE PROCESS OF CHANGE MODEL TO GRIEF

Our journey through what has been found to both hinder and help practitioners confronting complex grief may best be brought to life by revisiting the two cases introduced at the beginning of this chapter. Both are examples of complex grief within cultural context and involve family, professional contexts, and others. These cases are also excellent examples of how the process of change model integrates the combined recommendations of recent effective approaches to doing interventions with complex and complicated grief.

The Case of Hope

Recall that Hope was experiencing near psychotic symptoms following the tragic death of her cousin. She was losing sleep and missing work, and her son was acting up. She did not understand what was happening and came in for whatever help she could get.

Interventions with Hope followed all of the more recent recommendations for handling complicated and complex grief. They may best be summarized as follows:

- As far as the first step of forming a relationship with Hope, after learning the story of her cousin's death, the practitioner validated Hope's distress and experiences by validating and normalizing them, given her life and family traditions.

- The therapist and Hope discussed her distress over not even being able to say goodbye to her cousin and tell him how much he had meant to her.

- As a follow-up, the practitioner asked what Hope would say to her cousin if he was in the therapy room with her right now. They then did an empty chair exercise where she said what she needed to say to him in the alternate empty chair.

- The two of them talked about the gruesome nature of her cousin's death and the horror of seeing his face recreated in wax in the casket.

- Building on that experience, the practitioner also validated Hope's experience of seeing her face melting in her mirror reflection as a reaction to viewing her cousin's face recreated in wax and putting her experience in context of what many might experience. With some of the following interventions, her vision of her face melting gradually vanished.

- Turning to Hope's feeling of someone being outside her door and the visions of someone standing beside a casket in her room at night, the therapist reflected on the idea that it had something to do with her incomplete experiences with her cousin before his death, helping to make further meaning of those experiences. This offered both a rationale for her experiences and a potential pathway for her to resolve those experiences.

- Based on this discussion, Hope agreed to *invite* her cousin into her bedroom, at least figuratively, when she sensed a presence outside her door or the vision at night—a reversal of her previous avoidance. The practitioner also shared examples of others over the past who had very similar experiences, thus normalizing Hope's experience in the context of others who had similar intensely distressing losses. Hope followed this directive over several evenings, and she eventually found those experiences and visions to go away as she felt more comfortable and resolved with his loss. This returned a feeling of regained control and understanding of her experiences and moved her toward better resolution. This was a classic prescription to go toward the experiences rather than away from them.

- Agreeing that her son likely was aware of her distress and that of the family, Hope brought him into the consulting room and shared with him more of the details of her cousin's death and the related reasons for her own distress, thus also reversing her former pattern of trying to shield him from the death. To her surprise, her son said he had suspected this, and they hugged. Moving forward, his agitation gradually decreased.

- Eventually, Hope also brought her boyfriend in (he had to surrender his handgun at the front desk before joining them). Once more, to her surprise, after sharing more with him about her distress and grief, he shared his own similar distress following the death of an aunt who had raised him. He vowed to stay closer in the coming weeks to be a support.

- Hope also agreed eventually to call her sisters from the therapy office and talk to them about her experiences and learn of theirs. In response, they validated her distress and recounted their own. They offered to have Hope move in with them to share support and help more with her son. They also agreed to set more limits with their mother to keep her out of their affairs going forward. All were affirmed in their experiences as normal given the extreme situation of their cousin's death.

Hope and her boyfriend also began setting alarms for Hope to get up in the morning and began setting limits with her son as he acted up when she left for work. Her boyfriend and her sisters began taking turns watching him during the coming days. All of this occurred within the span of roughly 4–6 weeks—at which time, Hope was beyond all of her distressing experiences and she, her boyfriend, and her sisters agreed that their lives had, in fact, moved more positively than they had ever been before the tragedy.

All of these interventions included validating, normalizing, and prescribing, as discussed in Part I relating to the process of change model. They also followed the revised dual process model discussed earlier, as Hope deliberately oscillated, along with her boyfriend and sisters, through both loss-related and restoration-related experiences. They agreed that they had all been through a lot together and had a lot of joint grieving to do as they put their lives back together. Furthermore, all involved eventually moved forward within a set of life arrangements and experiences far exceeding where they had been before, as another example of posttraumatic growth.

The Case of Mr. C

In the case of Mr. C, culture, acculturation, religion, intergenerational interaction, and the medical–psychiatric setting came together to form a potentially dangerous intersection for all involved. Recall that Mr. C was a 75-year-old Korean American man who had recently experienced the death of his wife. He tried to tell his family he was okay, but he was becoming more forgetful and he even had experienced his wife's voice reassuring him. Mr. C, in fact, was dangerously close to another psychiatric hospitalization. If the current context and interactions were not shifted, the hospitalization and other adverse events were likely to happen.

Following the process of change model, Mr. C and his family took several more positive turns in their interactions at this tipping point connection with the practitioner. The interventions in this case were as follows:

- In the process of forming a relationship, meeting individually with Mr. C and hearing of the loss of his beloved wife, the practitioner validated and supported Mr. C in his grief. This may have been the first time Mr. C had someone support, understand, and validate the depth of his loss.

- His experience of hearing his wife's voice telling him she was okay and in the presence of Jesus was normalized and affirmed by the practitioner as offering the comfort that it had.

- Furthermore, Mr. C shared with the therapist that all the things his wife had done to manage their daily life were simply foreign to him, and at times beyond him as he felt heavy with his grief. This normalized Mr. C's experiences in the context of such a major life transition.

- The practitioner also validated Mr. C's anger with his son and family at their constant intrusions, calls, and visits where they seemed not to understand the depth of his loss. Mr. C then went on to discuss with the therapist how to get that to change. This aligned with Mr. C's values to be seen as still capable and his goal of having his family understand his grief at the loss of their mother and his cherished wife. It also reaffirmed his position in the family as its elder.

- Mr. C's son was then seen on his own. He entered into a long discussion of his concerns about his father, followed by discussing the nature of grief in an older man who has lost his lifelong companion. The practitioner and Mr. C's son also discussed his dad's resilience in coming to a new country, learning a new language, and raising a family. The practitioner asked if he as a son, along with his wife, might visit Mr. C a bit more regularly and share the sadness of losing his mother along with remembering all the good times they had over the years. In addition, the practitioner asked the son if he could ease up on calling his dad a bit to give his dad a chance to reach out to him, and he agreed. This contextualized and normalized his father's life and reactions, while then prescribing a reversal in how the son and his wife would share their grief and affirm that of their father.

- The therapist then shared with Mr. C the discussion with his son. The practitioner then asked Mr. C if he was open to having time with his son and his daughter-in-law to simply share their sadness over the passing of their mother and his wife. The therapist also asked if Mr. C would simply call his son a time or two each week to check in and give him an update on how he was doing—both clear reversals of their former patterns. His daughter-in-law also volunteered to come once a week to help Mr. C with some of the household chores and make up some meals for him to have over the week.

- Mr. C and the therapist then called his minister in the local Korean Christian church to let him know of Mr. C's need for some spiritual guidance and company. The minister readily agreed.

Over the following month, Mr. C felt greater affirmation and support from his family around their loss, and he also felt embraced and affirmed by his church. His son was also pleasantly surprised by his father's calls, and everyone dropped their worries about another psychotic break and potential hospitalization, including the medical staff—both products of contextualizing and normalizing Mr. C's grief.

The language used initially to describe Mr. C's case in the earlier description of when he first came to see the practitioner was purposefully put into the language of the medical and psychiatric community. This was done because this was the lens most likely to have been used in the past when Mr. C was brought in for help. When viewed through this psychiatric lens alone, Mr. C's "symptoms" and behavior now and in the past were most likely viewed as indicative of a psychiatric break—and this is not to say that he may not have gone through something like that in the past. (This overpathologizing from a medical model is also reflected in the potential for Hope in the first case to have been hospitalized due to her hallucinations and delusions.) However, when put in the context of Mr. C's Korean culture of origin, his religious affiliation with the Korean Christian church, his age, and the loss on his lifelong companion, all of his current reactions around his wife's death become very understandable. (Context most always makes sense of behavior, particularly in grief and mourning.) Not only was hospitalization averted, but it may not ever have been needed in the past had intervenors attended better to Mr. C's cultural context and the intensity of his experiences. The literature around ethnicity, expressed emotion, and schizophrenia in the life of chronically psychotic people shows that decreasing escalating vicious cycles of emotional interchanges in families is highly correlated with avoiding rehospitalization (Weisman et al., 2006).

Once more, this case included validation, normalization, and prescription. It included deliberate prescriptions that the family share both sad and positive emotions and memories around the loss. It literally *reversed* the interchanges between Mr. C and his son from his son's worried calls to his dad to Mr. C's unsolicited check-in calls to his son. It honored Mr. C's faith and culture and included a helpful other in his minister through his grieving. In sum, it operated within the multiple contexts of this case to not only resolve the case and avert a potential rehospitalization but also to initiate a new more positive path for all going forward.

The cases of Hope and Mr. C are both prime examples of how the process of change model flexibly incorporated the majority of what is now recommended for intervening in complex and complicated grief. We turn now to the final section, "Following the Process," to track our journey through the crisis of death and mourning.

FOLLOWING THE PROCESS

As with prior chapters, we close this chapter on crisis intervention in grief and mourning with some key takeaways.

- First is the clear finding that not all grief needs intervention, and that sometimes unsolicited, one-size-fits-all intervention can do more harm than good.

- Next, complicated or complex grief is likely the true target of intervention that has been shown to be effective.

- Also, true to the process of change perspective, such complicated grief may best be identified by rigid, repetitive, and longer-standing vicious cycles of (a) overinvestment in loss-oriented reactions while denying resolution-oriented activities or (b) overinvestment in restoration-oriented activities while denying the loss (or both) through oscillating cycles through grief and restoration.

- Practitioner interventions should target interdicting and redirecting those vicious cycles while honoring and engaging the language, culture, and context of those involved.

- Practitioners need to be sure to situate grief in its cultural and faith-based contexts.

- In most cases, it is best to normalize, validate, and simply be with those who grieve when the grief appears not to be complex or complicated. Practitioners, friends, and family should only engage in interventions around grief when people ask for such help. Complicated or complex grief is the target of intervention.

- Practitioners need to be sure to fit their language, frames, and validation only to those who are requesting help.

- Therapists should validate their clients' distress while helping them to find meaning in their loss within their clients' own context, language, and faith traditions.

- Practitioners should attend to the patterns of survivors' grief resolution, locating any rigid ruminating sadness or exclusive denial and reconstruction efforts.

- Therapists should prescribe oscillating survivors time to move deliberately between grieving loss-oriented time, restoration-oriented time, and adding recuperation time if there have been multiple stressors and losses, to eventually strive for the survivor's sense of balance.

- When survivors or their social network (or both) seek help and when telltale rigidity and vicious cycles become apparent, a sensitive application of a variation of the dual process model in the process of helping all involved make more meaning of the loss. Shifting their vicious cycles of solution-generated problems and problem-generated systems holds the best promise of moving all toward more satisfying growth in their lives as they move forward.

- Finally, practitioners should remain open to and support all potentially transformative experiences that may evolve from all loss to help foster and support potential posttraumatic growth.

8 INTIMATE PARTNER VIOLENCE

Time-Limited Windows of Opportunity

Recall the case of Linda[1] from Chapter 4. Linda came in with her husband, Chuck, who had called a few days earlier saying he needed to find out why he was getting so violent with his wife. We saw Chuck alone first, in that he was the requesting client, then we saw Linda alone. There had been an escalating cycle of domestic violence over the past year, increasing in severity and frequency, along with growing isolation of the couple, especially Linda, from others. Chuck told of a history of having been robbed and hit over the head, using medication for a bad back, and having a habit of consuming beer and other alcohol. He wondered if those were the reasons for his violence. Linda came in with two swollen, seeping, black eyes, holding her painful ribs after a violent argument days earlier. She told Chuck to get help or she might need to leave him, and that was why they were here. She also loved Chuck and simply wanted to help him. She thought he had broken her arm earlier but was too embarrassed to seek medical help. Others told her to leave Chuck, but she wanted to have someone help her to stay if she could.

---

[1]All case examples are based on real clients, whose identities have been disguised to maintain confidentiality.

https://doi.org/10.1037/0000445-009
Crisis Intervention: Using Tipping Points to Achieve Transformative Change in Therapy, by J. S. Fraser

INTIMATE PARTNER VIOLENCE AS AN ENDEMIC CRISIS

Linda's case encompasses most of the typical elements of intimate partner violence (IPV). We will return to this case twice in this chapter: once to demonstrate the classic components of IPV, and again to discuss using an initial contact as a window of opportunity to initiate a new potentially virtuous cycle out of a repeated cycle of violence. IPV (like sexual assault and rape, which will be covered in the next chapter) is an endemic crisis. That is, IPV is a product of the cultural context that shapes it. Rigidly defined gender roles, cultural norms, religious beliefs and values, and defined differences in power, privilege, and control, among other factors, shape consequent interpersonal patterns. Recalling the three-sphere process of change working diagram of the therapy contract from Part I (Figure 4.2), IPV is shaped by the cultural context sphere. There are thus two levels for intervention in endemic crises such as this. The first level is to attempt to reshape the language, norms, and laws of the *cultural context* to gradually shift their influence over how this context shapes IPV. The second level is that of direct clinical interventions with either victims/survivors or perpetrators of violence. The second level addresses both the client and therapist spheres with interventions aimed at interdicting and redirecting the perpetrator's violence and shifting the victim/survivor's position on the violence while intervening to reduce its subsequent harm. This chapter will therefore follow that approach and discuss IPV in two parts. First, we will define IPV, describe its incidence, and give a brief history of how its visibility has been raised culturally. Then we will turn to interventions.

INTIMATE PARTNER VIOLENCE IN CONTEXT

As IPV is an endemic crisis, it is important to put it in context. In this section, we will describe how IPV has been referred to by different terms, discuss its incidence in the United States and globally, and provide a brief history of how IPV has gained attention within culture generally.

Defining the Problem and Its Scope

Although earlier descriptions of violence between intimate partners often used the terms *wife battering*, *domestic violence*, and others, the realization that similar violence occurs in same-sex relationships, courting and dating relationships, and other diverse partnerships has led to the use of the broader and now common term *intimate partner violence* (Walker, 2006). According to the National Center on Domestic Violence, Trauma, and Mental Health, "The term IPV refers to an ongoing pattern of coercive control maintained through physical, psychological, sexual, and/or economic abuse that varied in severity and chronicity" (Warshaw et al., 2013). Snead et al. (2018) offered a more thorough definition:

> IPV is defined as physical, sexual, or psychological harm perpetrated by a current or former romantic partner which may include: *physical violence* as the intentional use of physical force that has potential to cause death, injury, or harm; *sexual violence* consisting of rape or penetration, nonphysically pressured unwanted penetration, unwanted sexual contact, and noncontact unwanted sexual experience; *psychological aggression* such as the use of verbal or nonverbal communication with the intent to harm another person mentally or emotionally; and/or *stalking*, characterized by a pattern of repeated, unwanted attention and contact that causes fear or concern for one's safety. (p. 269, italics in the original)

Incidence of Intimate Partner Violence

Next, we will discuss the incidence of IPV in the United States and globally. We also note how this incidence is being broadened to include different genders and relationships.

Intimate Partner Violence in the United States

The 2015 National Intimate Partner and Sexual Violence Survey reported that approximately 35.4% of U.S. women had experienced IPV in the form of rape, physical violence, or stalking at some point in their lifetime. Of those women, 30.6% had experienced physical intimate violence, 21% had experienced severe violence, and 29.1% had experienced slapping, pushing, and shoving (Smith et al., 2018). Estimates range from one in four to one in three U.S. women having experienced IPV in their lifetime. These stark figures are likely underestimates of the extent of IPV for a wide range of reasons, including fear of retribution, embarrassment, lack of options and resources, and isolation from others, among myriad other obstacles to reporting.

According to the 2010 National Intimate Partner and Sexual Violence Survey conducted by the U.S. Centers for Disease Control and Prevention (CDC), "Among women who experienced rape, physical violence, and/or stalking in the context of an intimate relationship, the majority of bisexual and heterosexual women (89.5% and 98.7%, respectively) reported only male perpetrators" (Walters et al., 2011, p. 27). The study by Walters et al. provided strong evidence of the cultural context that supports male privilege and dominance in the culture at large. In essence, that context is termed the *patriarchy*, defined as "social organization marked by the supremacy of the father in the clan or family, the legal dependence of wives and children, and the reckoning of descent and inheritance in the male line" or "broadly: control by men of a disproportionately large share of power" (Merriam-Webster, n.d.-b). The feminist position on the force driving such domestic violence or IPV is power and control invested in male individuals through patriarchal cultural traditions. The more rigidly entrenched the cultural patriarchal beliefs and practices, the higher the likelihood of IPV toward women. Or, as we will see, it may be better said that violence flows from those with more power and control to those who do not have it, no matter the gender or relationship.

Intimate Partner Violence Globally

In a recent study, Sardinha et al. (2022) reported global, regional, and country estimates of IPV based on data from the World Health Organization Global Database on Prevalence of Violence Against Women. The investigators summarized the results as follows:

> Globally 27% of ever-partnered women aged 15–49 years are estimated to have experienced physical or sexual, or both, intimate partner violence at least once in their lifetime. However, there are variations by region of the world ranging from the highest in Oceania (49%; 38–61%) and central sub-Saharan Africa (44%; 33–55%), followed by Andean Latin America (38%; 31–46%) and eastern sub-Saharan Africa (38%; 31–44%). The prevalence of lifetime physical or sexual, or both, intimate partner violence was also high, and more than the global average, in south Asia (35%; 26–46%) and north Africa and the Middle East (31%; 24–40%). (Sardinha et al., 2022, p. 808)

Once again, these are stark figures attesting to the endemic nature of IPV around the world, with more traditional cultures in middle-income and low-income countries reporting some of the world's highest incidents of violence against women.

Broadening Incidence to Different Genders and Relationships

Lest we assume that IPV is purely a heterosexual phenomenon, a recent review of the literature on violence in same-sex couples noted the following:

> Lifetime prevalence of IPV in LGB couples appeared to be similar to or higher than in heterosexual ones: 61.1% of bisexual women, 43.8% of lesbian women, 37.3% of bisexual men, and 26.0% of homosexual men experienced IPV during their life, while 35.0% of heterosexual women and 29.0% of heterosexual men experienced IPV. (Rollè et al., 2018)

We will discuss issues around this gender focus next.

Moving From a Gender Focus to Power and Control

Although the feminist position asserts that male dominance and control is the driving force behind IPV, the data suggest that IPV goes beyond pure hetero-sexual partnerships. Newer thinking, however, suggests that there are multiple situated factors affecting *all* relationships aside from gender or sexual orienta-tion alone. It may be that the influence of attempts to control *any* relationship through exerting power and control over one's partner are the most important factors. In their examination of differences in IPV outcome, Caldwell et al. (2012) stated the following:

> We argue that power, and the abuse of power in intimate relationships, is the central issue in explaining why IPV occurs and why outcomes of IPV are typi-cally more severe for women than for men. . . . Gender, then, serves as a proxy for power. We believe a fruitful area of future research is to explore the contex-tual factors that create and sustain power differences in relationships. (p. 53)

Further research is also needed on other status variables related to more or less power and privilege in a culture (race, socioeconomic status, immigration status, etc.), physical size and strength, and other factors such as economic power, attachment to a partner who is the only source of emotional support, lack of access to resources, lack of education, fear of losing the children, disability status, and so forth. These elements relate to the cultural and interpersonal context spheres in our process of change working diagram (Figure 4.2), all of which boil down to the influence of power and control in interpersonal relationships.

Over the years, the majority of attention as well as the professional litera-ture have focused on violence against women. This focus has been noted as a problem. In a review of research on the effectiveness of intervention programs for perpetrators and victims on intimate violence, Eckhardt et al. (2013) stated that "none of the 61 empirical studies included in this review included a single female-designated abuse perpetrator nor a single designated male abuse victim . . . including abuse in gay and lesbian relationships and female perpe-tration in heterosexual relationships" (p. 224). In another more recent system-atic review and meta-analysis, Micklitz et al. (2024) urged the following:

> [I]t is crucial that research and practice integrate survivors of all genders. Except studies evaluating couple interventions, no study included male or nonbinary people affected by IPV and only one study explicitly included trans women (Glass et al., 2022) despite comparable or increased prevalence of IPV in these populations compared to cis-women (McLeod et al., 2020). (pp. 1010–1011)

With this in mind, much of what can be said in this overview is constrained by approaches and programs addressing female individuals as victims/survivors and male individuals as perpetrators. We may assume that the broad influence of power and differences in control are likely to be found in these other populations as well. The jury is still out, however.

LEVEL 1: INTERVENTIONS IN INTIMATE PARTNER VIOLENCE AT THE CULTURAL LEVEL

As noted earlier, two levels of intervention are needed for endemic crises. The first level aims at changing the cultural context of language, norms, traditions, laws, and resources. What follows are several of the most important interventions that have moved the cultural context, albeit slowly. For the practitioner confronted with an IPV case in the office or community, this level of intervention may seem far from offering direction; however, in many ways, this level has been opening the door for practitioners to *do* more direct clinical intervention today.

Changing Laws

The hearings before the U.S. Commission on Civil Rights in 1979, the U.S. Attorney General's Task Force on Criminalization of Violence Against Women and Children in 1983, the U.S. Surgeon General's Report on Violence Against Women and Children in 1985, as well as hearings before different committees of the U.S. Congress in the 1980s and 1990s (Walker, 1999) are examples of efforts to change laws in the United States regarding violence against women. The Violence Against Women Act (VAWA) has been of ongoing interest to Congress since its enactment in 1994. The original VAWA was intended to change attitudes toward domestic violence, foster awareness of domestic violence, improve services and provisions for victims, and revise the manner in which the criminal justice system responds to domestic violence and sex crimes (Violence Against Women Act, 1994). In 1995, the Office on Violence Against Women was created administratively within the U.S. Department of Justice (DOJ) to administer federal grants authorized under the VAWA. In 2002, Congress codified the Office on Violence Against Women as a separate office within the DOJ. In February 2013, Congress passed legislation that reauthorized most of the programs under the VAWA, among other things (Violence Against Women Reauthorization Act, 2013). All of these efforts not only raised the visibility of domestic violence in the United States, they also created formal intolerance for such violence and considered it a criminal act appropriate for arrest and prosecution. In general, both nationally and internationally, violence against women has been viewed as gender based, and this feminist perspective that is accepted across the world, where women and girls are seen as targets of male abuse, is likely a product of gender-based socialization or the patriarchy (Walker, 1999).

The Shelter Movement

As with the sexual assault movement covered in the next chapter, the domestic violence shelter movement began in the late 1960s and 1970s as a product of cultural consciousness-raising efforts around abuse of women. The original safe houses were located in apartments and homes as safe havens for women who needed to escape their abusers. They were spurred on by the VAWA of 1994 and its renewals since then with provisions of partial funding and mandates for interagency collaboration. In their review of shelters, Messing et al. (2015) noted, "Today, shelters remain the primary entry point for services such as emergency and transitional housing, therapy and support groups, advocacy for the attainment of resources, and legal advocacy; shelters also commonly house crisis hotlines" (p. 307). Messing et al. also recounted data from a national census of domestic violence services showing that "domestic violence agencies served 66,581 survivors in a single day in 2013 [and] on that same day, 20,267 hotline calls were answered" (p. 307). Shelters have moved to augment funding through collaborations with law enforcement, yet both national trends and these legal linkages have moved many services from victim-centered services to perpetrator-centered services. This shift in services came despite some earlier meta-analyses of 10 randomized controlled studies (Ramsay et al., 2009) reporting that advocacy interventions, increased social support, and women's use of safety planning and services decreased violence at 12- to 24-month follow-up. Messing et al. (2015) agreed and noted the following:

> advocacy and empowerment have been considered best practices in domestic violence intervention since the movement's inception, and women who feel more control over the process are generally more satisfied. [Yet] [p]roviding women with tangible resources that allow them to become self-sufficient—such as well-paid employment and childcare—may be more powerful than advocacy alone (Rollins et al., 2012). (p. 308)

Provision of support, advocacy, and housing options thus appears to be a major contributing factor to the ongoing success of domestic violence shelters both in the United States and internationally. Yet the criminal justice response to IPV has also increased, and this response became better funded and a resource for support of the shelter and domestic violence movement in general. A byproduct of this shift has been an emphasis on perpetrator arrests and treatment for perpetrators at times at the expense of supporting victim/ survivor services. To understand this cultural-level effect on survivors, and particularly on the mandatory arrest and treatment of perpetrators, we now turn to the impact of the Duluth model.

The Impact of the Duluth Model

Barner and Carney (2011) described the influential Duluth model and its inception as follows:

> The psycho-educational treatment approach for perpetrators of IPV originated by the Duluth Domestic Abuse Intervention Project (DAIP), commonly referred to as the Duluth model, began in 1981 with a multi-institutional team of emergency responders (i.e., 911 operators), police departments, prosecutors, courts, several existing women's shelters, and human service agencies. (p. 237)

They continued:

> The model, in its initial stages, showed significant successes, and, as Pence and Paymar (1993) have noted, collaboration on this level seemed to provide for the mandates and needs of all of the institutions and soon drew the attention of the national law enforcement bodies, women's rights groups, and others who encouraged its replication in other cities. Advocates of the Duluth model also proved adept at lobbying for legislative changes to promote the adoption of the model, and "negotiate . . . agreement with the key intervening legal agencies to coordinate their interventions through a series of written policies and protocols" (Pence & Shepard, 1999) such as mandatory arrest laws, the first of which was successfully lobbied in Duluth, Minnesota by representatives of the DAIP. Within ten years of its founding, programs patterned on the Duluth model were the primary interventions for IPV in all fifty of the United States (Pence & Paymar, 1993). (Barner & Carney, 2011, p. 237)

A related and important note on the Duluth model was its psychological use of what it termed the *power and control wheel* and its desired alternative of an *equality wheel* describing qualities of relationships to be strived for (Pence & Paymar, 1993). The power and control wheel depicts a circle or wheel with power and control at its hub and the rim of physical and sexual violence around the outside. Eight spokes represent the following actions: (a) using intimidation; (b) using emotional abuse; (c) using isolation; (d) minimizing, denying, and blaming; (e) using children; (f) using male privilege; (g) using economic abuse; and (h) using coercion and threats. By contrast, the equality wheel has equality at its hub, nonviolence as its rim, and eight spokes representing the following: (a) nonthreatening behavior, (b) respect, (c) trust and support, (d) honesty and accountability, (e) responsible parenting, (f) shared responsibility, (g) economic partnership, and (h) negotiation and fairness. The fact that the elements of both wheels are so obviously face-valid and compelling has resulted in their use as a psychoeducational core for both female survivor groups and male perpetrator groups for decades across the United States. Later in this chapter, we will review both women's groups and perpetrators' groups using these power wheel psychoeducational tools.

Although the collaborative and integrated design of the Duluth model was and is admirable and useful, its advocacy for mandatory arrest based on the results of one preliminary study was flawed. As stated by Hoppe et al. (2020) in their more recent meta-analysis,

> [i]deally, a single study, such as the Minneapolis DV [domestic violence] experiment, should not be solely relied upon when making policy decisions. . . . Nevertheless, experimental results often are interpreted by policymakers as a correct test of policy and serve as evidence to support the adoption of policy. . . . Given the shift in public perceptions of DV as a police matter during the 1980's, law enforcement was eager to improve their response to DV and mandatory arrest policies were widely adopted following Sherman and Berk's (1984) initial study. (p. 4)

Hoppe et al. (2020) concluded as follows:

> The findings of the current meta-analysis are important because it offers support for the contention that arrest for DV-related offenses is largely ineffective in preventing or reducing repeat offending . . . [and at times] arrest for DV *may increase* the likelihood of repeat offending. (p. 16, italics in the original)

As can be seen here and in the next chapter on sexual assault, the cultural context sphere is highly resistant to change. This is not to diminish the overriding impact of multiple shifts in laws and provision of services. As noted in Part I of this book, in open process-based systems, change often moves gradually until it reaches a cliff of all-or-nothing change or a tipping point. For better or worse, the single study supporting the Duluth model (Sherman & Berk, 1984) was that tipping point.

LEVEL 2: DIRECT CLINICAL INTIMATE PARTNER VIOLENCE INTERVENTIONS

In their historical review of interventions for IPV, Barner and Carney (2011) concluded the following:

> Utilizing a historical review of interventions for IPV has shown several shifts and reversals in scope, focus, and treatment practices over time. Most significant is the historical reversal in the role played by the criminal justice system

in providing interventions for IPV, the reversal in dominance from a victim focus to a perpetrator-centric focus for IPV interventions, and the shift from a victim advocacy perspective to a coordinated community response paradigm. [However,] a review of the literature on mandatory arrest and prosecution laws and the behavioral intervention programs as part of the larger paradigm of coordinated community response suggests a lack of empirically supported practices in treatment for perpetrators and victims and inconclusive data on effectiveness of mandated or supported treatment modalities. (p. 242)

Thus, not all pattern reversals and shifts are differences that make a difference. Recall that most first-order solutions make complete sense to all involved, yet they do not always work and at times may make things worse. Let us take a closer look at the other two spheres of our process of change working diagram—client and practitioner—to see what guidance they offer practitioners as they encounter victims/survivors and perpetrators directly.

Practitioners need to be aware of the ongoing efforts to shift the cultural context of IPV, as reviewed in the previous section. The cultural elements that underlie IPV and the barriers to victims disclosing, much less following through with reporting and prosecution without encountering secondary victimization at the hands of those designated as helpers, are slowly shifting.

The impact of the Duluth model at the cultural context level has clearly overlapped with more direct clinical intervention. In that way, it formed a bridge between more general advocacy to change IPV laws and raise awareness within the general public regarding IPV and the beginning of more organized and focused interventions. Perhaps a closer look at how the Duluth model has influenced women's groups will shed more light on how it plays out.

Women's Groups

As a result of the overwhelming influence of the Duluth model throughout the United States, integrated programs for women who are victims of violence have proliferated. Furthermore, these programs have been infused with the feminist perspective that IPV is a direct result of the patriarchy, with a strong focus on power and control. Thus, the power and control wheel and the equality wheel have become a standard feature of groups both within shelters and in postshelter intervention. Groups use a psychoeducational format to develop changes via education and resocialization. It is not put forward as a therapeutic intervention. Personal empowerment has been a consistent theme linked with success for this approach. However, high dropout rates have been observed in both Duluth-oriented groups and in shelters in general. Therefore, the model itself is likely most effective for those who have been receptive to its message. Once more, we return to the theme that all interveners with clients in crisis need to attend to fitting a rationale that makes sense to their clients in order to go forward toward change. Failing this, clients will likely drop out and consequently stay stuck in their vicious cycles. Another alternative may be found in more direct social advocacy as a bridge from the level 1 social change discussed earlier.

Social Advocacy

Of equal and often more importance are the integrated advocacy services both within and outside of shelter services that are an integral element of the Duluth model. In a systematic review of IPV interventions, Trabold et al. (2020) concluded:

> The literature also suggests there is a hierarchy of needs, specifically meeting basic life needs (e.g., food, shelter) and safety are necessary before women are able to focus solely on emotional well-being or improved mental health outcomes through individual or group therapeutic approaches. (p. 10)

A concurrent review also supported the effect of social support, as Ogbe et al. (2020) concluded:

> There is good evidence of the effect of IPV interventions focused on improving access to social support through the use of advocates with strong linkages with community-based structures and networks, on better mental health outcomes of survivors . . . these interventions work better compared to other forms of IPV interventions. (p. 1)

Relating to the common economic distress accompanying the efforts of partners to prevent them from working, destroy their credit, and leave them with no viable economic or housing options, the recent Domestic Violence Housing First approach (Sullivan, Guerrero, et al., 2023; Sullivan, López-Zerón, et al., 2023; Sullivan, Simmons, et al., 2023) involves providing IPV survivors with mobile advocacy, flexible funding, or both, depending on individual needs. Although effective, this approach requires greatly increased funding. These integrated elements of an approach such as the Duluth model are difficult to divide from the basic psychoeducational format of the feminist-based approach of the Duluth-oriented groups for survivors, yet it is hard to deny that attention to basic needs for food, shelter, and safety will always precede any openness to more therapeutic or psychoeducational efforts.

Cognitive Behavior Therapy

Moving beyond the pure Duluth model's formats for women's groups, cognitive behavior therapy (CBT) has been an alternate approach to domestic violence groups for both women and men. CBT considers interpersonal partner violence as a learned behavior and focuses on changing what it considers faulty cognitions, beliefs, and emotions, while incorporating related new communication skills and emotion control techniques and supporting goal-directed action. An overview of therapeutic interventions in IPV (Condino et al., 2016) noted two main programs that represent specific variations of the CBT approach: namely, cognitive trauma therapy for battered women (CTT-BW; Kubany et al., 2003, 2004) and the Helping to Overcome PTSD Through Empowerment (HOPE) program (Johnson & Zlotnick, 2009). The CTT-BW and HOPE programs focus on *intervening in trauma* using education, stress management, exposure therapy, and restructuring of guilt and shame-related cognitions, while addressing safety issues, quality of life concerns, and postshelter goals. Although the CTT-BW and HOPE approaches needed more independent research team studies, both showed excellent effects in reducing PTSD symptoms, depression, and trauma-related guilt. Both approaches heavily relied on reversing experiential avoidance through exposure, recalling the main effective intervention models we reviewed in Chapter 6 on trauma. (This parallels the process view of prescribing reversals in vicious cycle solution patterns as key to resolution.) In truth, however, by all reports, these techniques dovetail with the power and control messages of the Duluth model; for all intents and purposes, the CBT and Duluth model approaches are merged in most applications. In most recent evaluations of interventions for both survivors and perpetrators, the CBT and Duluth model approaches are basically merged as complementary, so it is difficult to determine the independent effect of either approach. Their generalized effects on breaking IPV cycles have generally been welcome and positive.

In their review of overall therapeutic efficacy of domestic violence interventions, Hackett et al. (2016) concluded that most domestic violence intervention studies have found consistently positive and significant effects for reductions in external stress and increases in psychological adjustment, social adjustment, and family relations. Hackett et al. found that when treatment focused on safety, self-esteem, or career self-efficacy, the results were most consistently positive and significant.

Hackett et al. (2016) also noted that interventions *do not* affect reoccurrence of violence or return to the abusive partner. In the conclusions of their review of IPV, Trabold et al. (2020) stated, "However, continued contact and relations to the perpetrator appear to moderate the effect with significant implications on outcomes" (p. 11). In other words, violence is likely to recur and continue as long as partners stay together. Eckhardt et al. (2013) made an even more compelling point about the fallacy of assuming that survivor interventions will have significant effects on reducing future violence from the perpetrators, pointing out the following problem:

> [when] the intervention is expected to change the behavior of the abuse perpetrator, who is not directly receiving services, by changing the victim . . . these effects require a complex, two-stage process. First, the intervention must produce relevant proximal changes in the victim client. Second, these changes in the victim must in turn alter the behavior of the perpetrator. Thus, the efficacy of intervention can break down at either or both levels. (pp. 223–224)

Thus, even when direct interventions with survivors are successful in numerous ways, there is a very weak link with reduced revictimization if the partners remain together or there is no intervention or contact with the perpetrator (or both occur). Next, we turn to interventions with perpetrators.

Perpetrator Intervention

Perhaps the greatest influence of the widespread adoption of the Duluth model of IPV intervention has been on how it addresses perpetrators. Women's shelters had developed with groups and advocacy services, and the model soon standardized use of the power and control wheel and psychoeducational formats for those groups. Certainly, the integration and coordination of services from police, legal, medical, and social advocacy groups, along with the passage of new laws designating IPV as a crime, have had very positive effects on raising the visibility of IPV and coordinating response and intervention. However, along with criminalizing domestic violence came mandatory arrest, prosecution, and required batterers group attendance for perpetrators. As we have seen, the promise of mandatory arrest has not had the hoped-for results in reducing subsequent violence and arrests. Yet what about the influence of required batterers groups?

Batterers Groups

Most batterers groups essentially follow the psychoeducational, feminist-inspired model of the survivors groups for women described earlier. Batterers groups are not put forward as a therapeutic intervention. They target changes via education and resocialization, again focusing on the power and control of the equality wheel and on group discussion to shape their format. Also, in parallel with women's groups for survivors, batterers groups include strong CBT elements, including changing faulty cognitions, beliefs, and emotions while incorporating related new communication skills and emotion control techniques and supporting goal-directed action to stop violence and promote more egalitarian relationship skills.

Although there were high hopes for batterers groups, similar to the high hopes for mandatory arrest, these groups have been found to be *universally ineffective*. For example, in an overview of the research on batterers groups, Condino et al. (2016) stated the following:

> Overall, group treatments for IPV batterers have meagre effects on the cycle of violence. Most studies, regardless of intervention strategies (mandatory arrest, Duluth model group treatment, CBT), report that approximately one in three cases will have a new episode of IPV within 6 months based on the victim's reports. Moreover, this rate must be accepted with caution given the high attrition in victim reports across studies. (p. 83)

Soleymani et al. (2018) pointed to a wide range of problems with batterers groups, including high rates of nonattendance and treatment dropout, low motivation or readiness to change, problems in establishing a therapeutic alliance, and limited engagement in treatment activities. In other words, low motivation was consistently related to treatment dropout and reduced outcome across studies given mandatory referral to these groups. In a review of studies using motivational interviewing to match perpetrators' stage of change (i.e., precontemplative, contemplative, action oriented, or maintenance), Soleymani et al. found that the addition of motivational interviewing to batterers programs did not reduce future violence but did reduce dropouts and increase engagement.

Lack of effectiveness. *Survivor analysis* is a more sophisticated approach to studying failure in batterers group member outcomes. This analysis is used to examine the time between group completion and a new incident of violence—or provide a time-specific estimate of recidivism. Zarling et al. (2020) reported on a range of such studies and noted that several reported that the highest risk of domestic violence following intervention is within the first 100 days. Zarling et al. (2020) urged study of reoffence beyond the short term, noting the following:

> For example, Gondolf (2002) followed a sample of offenders referred to BIPs [batterer intervention programs] in three states over 4 years and found that recidivism rates increased over time from a little more than one third in the first 15 months from program assignment to nearly one half after 4 years. (p. 668; see also Gondolf, 2002, 2012).

Therefore, in the face of the widely acknowledged ineffectiveness of the widely adopted Duluth model and CBT groups for batterers, what might be the alternatives?

Returning to flexibility and fit. The need to change from a one-size-fits-all approach is broadly acknowledged across all therapy literature as well as in that addressing IPV (cf. Wampold & Imel, 2015). Snead et al. (2018) concluded their review of treatments that work for IPV by recommending that the "path to developing empirically supported treatments for domestic violence appears to require thinking outside the state-mandated box of men-only, feminist psychoeducational group interventions and tailoring the treatment to the individuals and couples devastated by domestic abuse" (p. 181). This view matches the process of change recommendations advocating for the idea of flexibility and fit between client and treatment and between client and therapist, and for the practitioners themselves (cf. Fraser, 2018; Norcross, 2002). Yet what might the options be? Soleymani et al. (2018) recommended the following:

> Given the association of therapeutic alliance to positive outcomes, a viable strategy for improving the success of IPV treatment may be to tailor treatment to maximize clients' agreement with the goals of intervention and trust in their therapists, as well as developing strategies that specifically address the perpetrator's motivation to engage in treatment. (p. 120)

All of these recommendations align with the basic positions of the process of change perspective. As we turn next to a more recent development in IPV interventions, we will note the initial effect of delivering an alternative treatment model that is closely aligned with most of the process of change premises and has held promise of at least equal if not better outcomes (Berta & Zarling, 2019; Zarling et al., 2019, 2020).

Achieving Change Through Values-Based Behavior

An acceptance and commitment therapy (ACT) approach for partner aggression (Berta & Zarling, 2019; Zarling & Berta, 2017; Zarling et al., 2020) has adapted the main premises and tactics of the ACT approach of Steven Hayes et al. (2012) to interventions with IPV. ACT is a third-wave therapy that builds on the cognitive behavior tradition, focusing on increasing psychological flexibility by promoting acceptance and mindfulness processes. This approach, Achieving Change Through Values-Based Behavior (ACTV), has been developed, piloted, tracked, and applied within a correctional system (in Iowa) as a protocol for conducting groups for convicted IPV offenders. The groups consist of 24 weekly sessions of 90 minutes each. They are open to new members during treatment and move through five phases, from big picture/core skills (seven sessions and revisited as needed) to emotion regulation skills (four sessions), cognitive skills (four sessions), behavioral skills (five sessions), and, finally, barriers to change (four sessions). Initial pilots used trained psychology doctoral students as facilitators, yet subsequent applications used trained corrections personnel as facilitators. A thorough review of this approach is beyond the scope of this chapter; however, a summary of its premises and interventions may help. In discussing the development of the ACTV approach, Zarling and Berta (2017) described its differences from prior approaches as follows:

> First, ACTV differs from other programs in the conceptualization of the causes of partner-aggressive behavior. In contrast to assumptions that aggression is an attempt to assert power over women (implicit in the Duluth model) or the result of angry thoughts and feelings (implicit in the CBT model), the ACT model of aggression is based on the premise that aggression has many possible causes and can only be fully understood "in context." By design, ACTV facilitators do not make a priori assumptions about the causes of any one person's violent behavior but rather encourage the offenders [to] notice and identify the antecedents and consequences of their own behavior while using their experiences as fodder for group discussion and skills training. This is consistent with the substantial evidence showing that men who engage in partner aggression represent a heterogeneous group, and, in turn, there is very little evidence to justify the practice of mandating all perpetrators to interventions assuming power and control issues are the cause of violence. (p. 99)

The ACTV approach begins by identifying group members' values and goals and then helping each member link those goals with actions that help them build toward those goals in their lives and relationships. The approach assumes that avoiding or attempting to control uncomfortable thoughts and feelings (termed *experiential avoidance*) only exacerbates those thoughts and feelings and contributes to interpersonal avoidance (a solution-generated vicious cycle similar to what we termed *mastery by avoidance* in our discussion of trauma in Chapter 5). The approach teaches skills to separate the links between group members' distressing thoughts and emotions and acting on them (termed *cognitive fusion and diffusion*). As Zarling and Berta (2017) explained,

> Overall, the ACTV program focuses on experiential learning of the ACT processes, building patterns of valued behavior, and addressing barriers to behavior change. The ACT processes are framed as skills that one can practice and learn, and these skills are practiced during group sessions. The overall goal is learning new ways to respond to cognitive and emotional experiences in a way that promotes effective, value-based living. (p. 95)

Mindfulness skills are taught to help decrease emotional distress and allow participants to stay in the present moment, become aware of their current thoughts and emotions, and match them with their values and goals if they choose to act on them. They seek to move participants from being rigidly guided by internal thoughts, feelings, and urges (termed *psychological inflexibility*) to engaging in valued patterns of activity in line with their goals and values independent of internal experiences such as anger, fear, and frustration (termed *psychological flexibility*). Group facilitators are also encouraged to practice collaboration and flexibility and to maintain a non-judgmental attitude matching that desired of group members. The reader may recognize that most of these positions parallel the process of change approach described in Part I of this volume.

Research on the Achieving Change Through Values-Based Behavior Approach

Some admirable research has been done on the ACTV approach. In early pilot work, Zarling et al. (2015) found that individuals who received a 12-week version of the intervention had significant decreases in physical and psychological aggression at 6 months posttreatment compared with a matched control group, yet significant dropouts were still noted. In an earlier, related study, these researchers found that compared with a Duluth/CBT group, the ACTV completers experienced one-half the rate of domestic assaults postintervention (Zarling et al., 2015). A more recent study conducted by an independent research team and using correctional officers as facilitators (Lawrence et al., 2021) provided additional evidence suggesting that the ACTV model may be more effective compared with a carefully matched comparison group using the Duluth/CBT-based model in a follow-up period of up to 5 years. Interestingly, in a further study of original research groups of the initial ACTV studies compared with the Duluth/CBT model that was extended out to 5 years using more sophisticated analyses (Zarling et al., 2020), several other elements were found. Although the ACTV groups rather consistently produced better recidivism results in shorter time periods, the final 5-year comparisons showed that both the ACTV and Duluth/CBT models converged to be relatively similar in their effectiveness. (This finding may reflect the position that using any organized rationale for treatment will likely have at least some impact on outcome; cf. Wampold & Imel, 2015.) Wampold and Imel also made an important point that there are likely some perpetrators who are more broadly subject to potential violence beyond IPV and account for most recidivism, and these men may need alternative interventions. Again, one size rarely fits all, and most bona fide and organized interventions produce better results than no treatment at all (Wampold & Imel, 2015; Wampold et al., 1997).

In summary, organized intervention groups with perpetrators have shown a similarly neutral to mildly successful level of effectiveness as those for women survivors of IPV. The only promising intervention with perpetrators adopts an approach very close to that of the process of change model advocated in this book. Specifically, it collaborates with perpetrators' ultimate values and goals, matches their current violent thoughts and actions with those values and goals, and then builds new, more fitting ideas and actions to achieve change in the violent patterns. This approach aligns with the process of change model, as we will see next in our discussion of how to intervene individually in the crisis of IPV.

THE PROCESS OF CHANGE AT TIPPING POINTS WITH INDIVIDUALS

Although efforts to alter components of the cultural context sphere in the process of change working diagram (Figure 4.2) have had significant impacts and efforts in the client and therapist spheres have focused on group interventions, this leaves us with a final consideration of how to proceed individually at the point of contact with intimate partners. Most intervenors, whether therapists or advocates, often encounter a battering relationship shortly after an incidence of violence; this is a tipping point to a window of opportunity for change. A therapist might also be confronted unexpectedly with spousal violence in a couple participating in therapy. Such surprises usually occur because the therapist has either not attended to existing patterns that may have predicted the violence or has so consistently seen the couple together that their common processes of colluded secrecy, intimidation, and protection have disguised the situation.

Nevertheless, whenever such a violent incident presents itself, direct action is called for. A crisis such as IPV is both a danger and an opportunity for the system members as well as for the therapist, so all must proceed with caution. For the victim/survivor, the danger of the incident lies in the possibility of future repeated violence. Its opportunity lies in the limited time during which the couple has increased motivation to end the fear and pain of violence and find new options. For the perpetrator, the danger lies in an increased loss of control, arrest, or the potential loss of the partner (or all three). Its opportunity lies in limiting the increasingly ineffective use of violence and opening new, safer, and more effective interactions. For the therapist, the danger lies in the responsibility to ensure the current and future safety of the victim/survivor while not alienating either partner from help. Its opportunity lies in the increased yet time-limited ability to access a dangerous, semiclosed system and help move it toward more openness and safety.

If the practitioner's goal is to alter or reshape the couple's interaction from within rather than to serve as a representative of strong social sanctions from without, then direct confrontation only undercuts this goal by producing immediate alienation. Initially, the therapist may be more able to disqualify the violence by not challenging it, or at least by not sanctioning it. As the intervention proceeds, the violence may then be disqualified gradually as too dangerous an option for either partner, as not as useful as other options, or as running counter to other goals or values of either partner. This is a sensitive issue. Although it is tempting for the practitioner to revile the violence, this stance may not only reduce the intervenor's options to eliminate it but also may, in some instances, escalate its potential and further close the system to future help.

From the process of change view, the major thrust is to identify, adopt, and use inherent system forces and channel them toward new and more desired ends. In this process, insidious cycles and patterns that have historically led to greater closure and increased potential for violence are directed instead toward increased openness and safety (cf. McCloskey & Fraser, 1997).

The primary goals of the process of change perspective are to (a) decrease isolation, (b) equalize power differentials, (c) disqualify violence as an accepted option, (d) increase the survivor's perception of self-control, and (e) increase the perpetrator's acceptance of responsibility for their actions while offering them new options. Each of these goals is a *pattern reversal* in the broad, vicious cycles of the generic patterns of IPV. Consequently, each of these goals and reversals is likely to feel counterintuitive to those involved. It is therefore crucial for practitioners to fit frames and therapeutic rationales to their interventions to help these reversals make sense to all involved. To these ends, it is important for the intervenor to be aware of both the common patterns that generally contribute to increasing closure and violence and the unique positions, ideas, and patterns of each relationship encountered.

Turning to more direct individual clinical intervention with IPV survivors and perpetrators, the process of change model incorporates the full range of the perspectives and practices reviewed earlier. A set of important elements of the process of change perspective on intervention is to be aware of any *generic patterns* or *solution-generated problems* around each crisis, and then remain open to all unique or specific variations. Then the main interventions revolve around understanding the values, goals, language, and culture that shape the survivor's attempts to deal with the aftermath of the repeated violence or the perpetrator's anger and attempts to lash out and control. The final steps are to track the vicious cycles around their situation, design interventions to interdict and reverse those patterns, and then support the pattern shifts once they begin.

In service of describing individual-level interventions, the next section will first address what has been called "battered woman's syndrome" as a potential generic pattern and then review the critiques of that concept. We will then track how these sets of interventions align with the general process of change model as it weaves its way through this pressing crisis. Finally, we will revisit the original case of Chuck and Linda to track how an intervention team intervened in this case using the process of change model to take advantage of the window of opportunity it presented.

Battered Woman's Syndrome as a Potential Generic Pattern

As if the layers of barriers to change described earlier are not enough for victims/survivors in IPV relationships, there is also the classic "battered woman cycle" model that may further draw women (in this case) into the relationship. (As noted earlier, there has been little attention or research on survivors or perpetrators of different genders or in same-sex relationships, for example. Once more, much of the attention has been focused on female victims and male perpetrators.) Perhaps no other writer, researcher, and advocate has had more influence on the area of IPV than Lenore Walker (1999, 2006, 2009). From her original research designed in 1978 in which she analyzed incidents from each of 400 subjects in more than 1,600 battering incidents, a pattern of violence was found matching a cycle of violence. This cycle of violence perspective has been sustained in the literature and is widely used today. In her description of that research, Walker (2006) stated the following:

> The pattern consisted of the initial courtship period followed by three phases that repeated themselves in a cycle. The first phase was named the *tension-building* phase where the perception of danger from the batterer kept escalating at different rates for different people. The battered woman tried to please the man during this period and her behavior could slow down or speed up movement into the second phase, or the *acute battering incident*. The second is the shortest part of the cycle but has the highest risk for physical or sexual damage. The third phase was called the period of *loving contrition*. During it, the batterer apologized and engaged in loving behavior. In some relationships, there was no loving behavior that could be recognized but the third phase was characterized only by a decrease or temporary cessation in the violence. (pp. 145–146, italics in the original)

Walker's initial explanation of the battered woman syndrome used the *learned helplessness* research of Maier and Seligman (1976). That series of studies showed that, in both animals and humans, the inability to escape noncontingent punishment resulted in complacency and even reluctance to escape, even when the opportunity presented itself. Walker's work also referred to the so-called Stockholm syndrome. The term *Stockholm syndrome* was coined based on a failed 1973 bank heist in Stockholm, Sweden, where the captives developed intimate bonds with their captors. Graham et al. (1995) conceptualized the syndrome based on four precursors necessary for its development: perceived threat to survival, perceived kindness, perceived isolation, and perceived inability to escape. All of these factors fit the cycle of violence traced by Walker. Pagelow (1984) paralleled the cycle pattern description, adding that there was a gradual process of growing isolation from others along with a growing incidence of severity from verbal abuse, to slapping and pushing, to punching and more. The cycle represents a downward spiral of continuing isolation and alienation from the outside world in a relationship marked by dominance and control. Over the years, this cycle has been clinically recognized and used to identify and intervene in a wide range of IPV relationships, and it is vividly apparent in the case of Linda and Chuck at the beginning of this chapter.

Chuck and Linda as a Prime Example

Chuck and Linda's case has all of the classic components of traditionally defined IPV. They each accept traditional gender roles, and there are great power differentials between them physically, socially, and economically. Their relationship is a semiclosed and closing system, which has increasingly isolated Linda from outside resources and limited the amount of information available to others about the two of them. They have cycled through the typical control-and-dominance cycle from gradual tension building, to violence, to a honeymoon phase, drawing them each in to begin another phase. As Linda said, "When he is about to beat me, seems like he says that I'm not good enough. Then, after he beats me, it's like ain't nobody can fill my shoes. . . . It's weird." Each cycle has gotten more severe and more frequent. Linda says, "He don't hit me with his hand no more. Now he beats me with his closed fists." Linda has moved into the classic learned helplessness and Stockholm syndrome positions. She fears the next battering and feels helpless to prevent it, yet she has a strong allegiance to her partner. She says, "I can feel it building. Like, I know what's going to happen. But knowing and knowing what to do about it are two different things."

Chuck, on the other hand, takes little responsibility for his actions, externalizing the reasons with numerous "bad habits" and external causes and stresses. It is likely that the main reason he has "come for help" is to appease his partner, but not necessarily to change. Outside others such as friends, family, or shelter advocates have been drawn into the dichotomous positions of advocating that Linda either adjust to the relationship or leave. Both of these positions only escalate the cycle.

Essentially, the attractor of the vicious cycle of violence draws others into well-meaning *power positions* with the victim/survivor as they tell her what to do. They become *beneficent perpetrators*, telling her how to deal with the violence or how to leave her perpetrating partner. As we described in Part I, others are drawn into a problem-generated system that risks further isolating the victim and perpetuating the vicious cycle of violence while paradoxically trying to be of help. This only tends to disempower the woman, disaffirms her feelings and position, creates further shame and guilt, and further isolates and alienates her from others, further emphasizing her helplessness and hopelessness. All involved are trying to manage risks and recreate stability, and their very actions are further feeding the attractor of the battering cycle. When this happens, all involved paradoxically perpetuate the very things they seek to change. Linda and Chuck's relationship seems to fit Walker's cycle of violence, reflecting a classic generic pattern.

Critiques of the Battered Woman's Syndrome

Lest we assume that Walker's (2006) battered woman's syndrome is without problems, there have been numerous critiques of it in recent years. First, from the feminist perspective and a contextual position, describing the cycle pattern as a "syndrome" tends to pathologize it rather than understand it as a response to a violent and power-dominant relationship. Still others are concerned about the notion that the survivor becomes helpless in the learned helplessness model. As Messing et al. (2015) concluded,

> as practitioners seek to empower clients toward safety, they should take into account the factors affecting women's choice to sever or remain in their relationship and the many ways they are connected to their partners (for example, love, finances, children). . . . Victim-survivors of IPV do not choose their abuse—they want it to stop, but may want alternatives to leaving their relationship or staying in a shelter. (p. 310)

Others address the fact that battered women's syndrome is based on heterosexual partnerships and does not allow space for LGBTQ+ relationships. In 1996, the DOJ ultimately rejected Walker's syndrome terminology, saying it did not have the support needed for a diagnostic category (Barner & Carney, 2011; Rothenberg, 2003; Walker, 2006). Power and control seem to be the common factor across all various intimately violent partnerships; therefore, this feminist perspective strives to achieve egalitarian and collaborative relationships as a better alternative. (Yet, it is important to remember that not all people who conform to more traditional nonegalitarian gender and relationship roles end up in IPV relationships.)

ENGAGING THE PROCESS OF CHANGE MODEL FOR IPV

As promised at the beginning of this chapter and following what we have done in previous chapters, we now return to the case of Chuck and Linda to see how the process of change model was successfully applied with them at the tipping point of their first contact and then going forward.

Returning to Chuck and Linda as a Case in Point

In the initial intervention with Chuck and Linda, it was evident that the couple presented at the unique opening of their relationship during the immediate aftermath of a violent attack. They were in the honeymoon or loving contrition phase according to Walker's (2006) cycle of violence view. The tasks were to assess the pattern; align with the language, positions, values, and goals of both parties; and initiate a process to begin to open their relationship while beginning an empowerment process with Linda and having Chuck initiate ownership for his violent actions.

Relationship Establishment

The practitioner met first with Chuck and empathized with his dilemma of repeatedly losing his temper and lashing out violently at his wife, Linda. His values and related goals were to understand why he was becoming violent and to find other alternatives so he did not lose his wife.

We then met with Linda and empathized with her pain and obvious injuries. We aligned with her goals to stay in the relationship if she could and to help Chuck see what his violence was doing to her so he would stop.

Information Gathering

The practitioner found that Chuck realized he was getting more violent and severe in his frustration and beatings of Linda. Chuck also offered multiple external reasons for not taking responsibility for his violence, including his alcohol use, the drugs he took for his pain, and how his pain shortened his temper. He described blacking out at one point in the most recent violent incident and then coming back to consciousness after beating Linda and finding blood on his hands. He was taking no personal responsibility.

Linda described a growing cycle of Chuck getting more violent and doing so more frequently. She also said she and Chuck were very close and she felt isolated from others. When others did learn of the violence, they all told her to leave, but that was not what she wanted.

Consensual Problem Formation, Goal Setting, and Treatment Planning

With Chuck, the practitioner agreed to collaborate in identifying the cause of his violence and helping find better alternatives. The practitioner aligned with Chuck's frame for the present that there might be an external cause and, if not, stated that they would look into better options for him.

With Linda, the practitioner agreed with her wish to help Chuck see what he was doing to Linda when he beat her and then change as a result of it.

Break/Recess for Processing

It was clear that the practitioner needed to let Linda know that the cycles going on between her and Chuck were very similar to an IPV pattern—yet not press her to leave but just observe. The idea was to see whether Linda would be willing to go with Chuck to the emergency room (ER), have her injuries attended to, and allow him to see the extent of what he had done. If Chuck was to be subsequently hospitalized for diagnostic reasons, then the practitioner wanted to see whether Linda was willing to stay with family or friends during his hospitalization.

With Chuck, the idea was to see whether the practitioner could reach out to Chuck's physician and collaborate with an inpatient admission to evaluate the extent of his head injury and the effects of the prescribed medications. It would also be important to allow Chuck to feel in control of the idea of having Linda go to the ER for her injuries and of him to accompanying her. It would also be important for Chuck to ask Linda about going to the ER in front of the practitioner.

Problem Solving and Interventions

The practitioner began by positioning with Linda to begin the process of empowering her. She was complimented for her strength, not only for coming in but also for sharing the details of the recent battering incident. To reinforce Linda's first steps to retake choice and control, the practitioner asked her how she had found the strength and courage to come in, share her situation, and make her wishes and needs known. The practitioner told her that going down to the first floor of the hospital to the ER and having Chuck with her to see her injuries might be the first step in having Chuck learn what he was doing to her—at the same time, it would allow the ER physician to assess her injuries. Although this option was offered as purely Linda's choice to make, it seemed in line with her goal of having Chuck see the impact of his violent attacks. Linda agreed but said she needed to have Chuck tell her directly that this was okay. It was agreed that Chuck would ask her to go to the ER while they were in session.

The practitioner told Chuck there was a way to get to the bottom of what might be making him more violent if anything was doing so externally. That is, they would collaborate with Chuck's primary care physician and have him admitted to the mental health inpatient unit "for tests and follow-up." Chuck agreed with the therapist that Linda might need attention to her current injuries. Chuck therefore agreed to accompany Linda to the ER and stay by her side. He also agreed to ask her to go to the ER with the practitioner present before the session ended.

Summary and Closure

In a final brief segment, the couple was seen together and the therapist affirmed their goals and explained the utility of going to the ER. Conveniently, the crisis staff worked regularly with the hospital ER staff (they were in the same hospital, four floors above the ER). When the couple agreed, the practitioner called the ER staff directly, explained the situation, and got agreement for Chuck to be in the examination room while they described to him the extent of Linda's injuries. The couple was then sent directly to the ER, and the ER staff was asked to confirm their arrival with a call back to the practitioner.

Shortly thereafter, the practitioner arranged for Chuck's hospitalization, during which time Linda went to live with family. The reasons for Chuck's violence were gradually ruled out while he was in the hospital, and he was then left with the task of taking more responsibility for his own actions. He was subsequently referred to a batterers group. Linda asked that the therapist not disclose her living situation to Chuck while she sorted her situation out with the practitioner and her family. She eventually entered a women's group. Although the couple did return to each other, they eventually separated and divorced, though they maintained contact with the therapist, their collaborative advocate, throughout.

Although this is just one unique case, it demonstrates a number of points we have emphasized in taking advantage of the tipping point when a couple enters a session around a recent incident of IPV. The couple was entering Walker's respite or honeymoon phase of the domestic violence cycle. As such, the perpetrator was likely to collaborate with the practitioner more to prove his contrition to his wife. The values and goals of both partners were validated and enlisted in a rationale to begin changing the violent cycle according to ways they both agreed would help. The survivor in this case was empowered by the practitioner complimenting her courage and aligning with the goals she set. The system was opened not only to the practitioner but also to the ER staff, the inpatient staff, and the survivor's family. Support was provided to the survivor through a women's group, and the perpetrator's external excuses for his violent behavior were taken away in collaboration with the inpatient staff. He was linked with a batterers group but soon dropped out. Once more, this was just one example of embracing the window of opportunity of a first session to enter a violent cycle and initiate a set of changes that likely would not have made sense or have occurred previously. Often, simple new triggers at such tipping points can initiate new positive virtuous cycles.

REVERSING PATTERNS IN IPV

Culturally, IPV has historically been kept out of public view as a more personal matter between partners. Typically, both guilt and shame have been associated with IPV. As we have described in this chapter, IPV relationships tend to become semiclosed and closing systems that create isolation from other relationships, information, and resources. Victims/survivors thus tend to become disempowered with less influence and control in these relationships. They often experience blame and shame, because they are often accused of never being able to be enough or to do enough for their partners. From a process perspective, violence in these relationships becomes an endemic periodic crisis, which evolves through periodic cycles that escalate in intensity and frequency over time, taking on characteristic generic patterns given the nature of the context and culture within which the partners live.

Thus, generally, the goals of all interventions are to alter the cultural context supporting this endemic pattern of repeating crises while opening and redirecting the flow of the patterns in the relationship out of the downward spirals that characterize them. As we reviewed in this chapter, these goals are met with efforts to change at two levels—one culturally, and the other clinically. Once more, the target goals of both levels represent pattern reversals.

Culturally, the target goals are to end the silence around IPV by doing the following: opening discussion of it; labeling it as intolerable versus a desired norm; advocating for new laws, practices, and sanctions against it; and developing new safe options and social and economic supports for survivors of that violence. As we have seen, the results and impact of these efforts have been impressive, as they have reversed the implicit secrecy and acceptance of IPV as simply a norm within a culture. These efforts represent a set of vicious cycle pattern reversals at the cultural level.

At the second level of clinical intervention, the goals resonate with those at the cultural level in terms of interdicting and reversing the generic vicious cycle patterns of violence. With intimate partners, the intervention goals are as follows: to open the system to outside input and resources, to equalize power differentials, to externalize the perceived source and reasons for the violence from residing purely in the survivor to locate it in relation to the perpetrator and the norms of the relationship and the culture, to offer perspective to those involved regarding the patterns of the violence as it evolves and re-cycles, and to identify the values and goals of the partners involved and redirect their interactions to help them to attain these goals and live by them.

All of these goals for endemic crisis intervention in IPV are embodied in both cultural and clinical levels of intervention and in the process of change model we have tracked throughout this chapter. Practitioners will do well to embrace all of these goals at both levels of intervention as they go forward in their practice with clients involved in IPV.

FOLLOWING THE PROCESS

As an endemic crisis, IPV is shaped by its cultural context. In this chapter, we tracked the nature and incidence of IPV and then showed how cultural advocacy to change laws and to raise visibility of IPV has begun to shift that larger context and to alter the nature of IPV in the United States and globally. Two levels of intervention were reviewed. The first level addressed group interventions for victims/survivors and for perpetrators and tracked their rationales and the extent of their effectiveness. The second level was that of more direct individual clinical intervention. Here, we again traced the process of change model and applied it to a specific case. A final set of key points may help to capture the essence of this review of IPV as an endemic crisis and interventions for IPV.

- First and foremost, IPV is a product of the context and culture surrounding it.

- Although most attention has been paid to violence by men against women, more attention is needed toward same-sex partnerships, women as perpetrators, men as victims/survivors, and the LGBTQ+ population, among other populations and types of relationships.

- Most theory and practice have converged on an agreement that IPV is a product of issues of power and control, with violence going from those with more of both to those with less.

- While mandatory arrest has become popular nationwide, its effects on reducing future IPV have been found to be minimal.

- Both women's groups and men's groups for IPV have proven to be marginal in their effectiveness, despite their widespread popularity.

- Direct advocacy and provision of empowerment and resources for survivors has proven to be one of the most effective interventions.

- Newer approaches that identify and align with perpetrators' values and goals and then help them adjust their current and future actions to them have shown the most promise with this population.

- All practitioners need to take advantage of any point of contact as a time-limited window of opportunity to join, validate, and create the beginning of some shift in the pattern of violence.

- Practitioners need to identify and collaborate with the values, goals, and wishes of all involved and honor them.

- Practitioners need to become aware of the regional laws and area resources relating to services and interventions in IPV and be able to use them.

- Practitioners always need to be aware of the potential risk factors of further violence and attend to generic patterns such as the cycle of violence phases, locating the clients within that cycle.

- Practitioners need to attend to the cultural context within which the violence is occurring and honor that context while seeking to gradually shift its effects.

- Practitioners need to become aware of the barriers present to disclosing violence or considering leaving the relationship.

- Practitioners must become aware of the range of intervention models available for both batterers and survivors and consider which ones, if any, match with the clients involved.

- With victims/survivors, practitioners need to validate the pain and distress of the violence and *externalize* its source and responsibility as residing in the partner or perpetrator and *not* in the survivor.

- Practitioners need to use positioning with survivors by asking how they have managed to survive. Shifting language to referring to the client as a survivor rather than a victim helps to confirm this subtle shift to an empowered role.

- Practitioners need to offer as many choices as possible to the survivor to help with the empowerment process.

- And finally, practitioners need to keep the door open to recontact, no matter the reasons.

9

SEXUAL ASSAULT

Intervening in Culturally Shaped Crises

Consider the following U.S. news reports on sexual assault at a cultural level:

In April 2023, a New York jury heard graphic details about Donald Trump's alleged rape of former advice columnist E. Jean Carroll in a defamation trial brought by Carroll in a lawsuit against the former president (Schonfeld, 2024). After Carroll described the incident where Trump allegedly sexually assaulted her in a department store dressing room years earlier, she responded to defense questioning on why she had not said anything until now when she was filing suit for more recently being defamed publicly by Trump. She replied, "I didn't want to make a scene. I didn't want to make him angry at me. . . . I don't remember screaming," Carroll testified. "I'm not a screamer. I'm a fighter," she said. Carroll testified that she confided in two friends and received conflicting advice—go to the police or don't, because Trump could use his wealth to harm her reputation. Carroll did not file a police report or a lawsuit until 2019, when she filed the defamation lawsuit. Trump was eventually found guilty of battery and defamation and fined $83.3 million. The case is under appeal at this writing.

Now consider this incident:

In 2022, Harvey Weinstein (a powerful American film producer) faced sexual assault charges in court (Reuters, 2024). They were brought by a foreign

https://doi.org/10.1037/0000445-010
Crisis Intervention: Using Tipping Points to Achieve Transformative Change in Therapy, by J. S. Fraser

model and actress whose account was corroborated by the testimony of others claiming similar sexual assaults at his hands. The trial was viewed by many as a partial consequence of the #MeToo movement (to be discussed in this chapter). After the actress described the assault in her hotel room some time earlier, she told the court she had not come forward with her allegations before this because she feared for her safety and that of her children in the face of Weinstein's power in the film industry. Weinstein's conviction in New York, and sentencing of 23 years in prison, was eventually overturned on appeal because the judge had allowed other women not directly involved in the case to testify. Some decried the verdict being overturned as another reflection of a judicial system out of touch with procedures allowing testimony on the extent of powerful perpetrators' patterns of assault. As of this writing, the case awaits a retrial in New York.

Finally, consider this incident:

> On January 18, 2015, 22-year-old Chanel Miller was sexually assaulted behind a dumpster on the Stanford University campus by Brock Turner, a 19-year-old star Stanford swimmer (Gersen, 2023). Two male graduate students noticed the assault in progress and held Turner down until the police arrived. The case made national news as it went to trial. Turner was eventually convicted of three felony sexual assault charges and sentenced to 6 months in jail followed by 3 years of probation when the trial concluded in March 2016. After serving half of his sentence, Turner was released for good behavior 3 months later. Four years later, Chanel Miller ended her anonymity in the case as its victim and stepped forward as a survivor, as she recounted her story in the book, *Know My Name: A Memoir* (Miller, 2020).

These incidents represent *cultural-level context* issues surrounding the identification and response to sexual assault, and they also describe a movement in U.S. culture to begin sanctioning perpetrators, continued challenges for victims/survivors, and struggles in the court system with applying consequences. In an upcoming section of this chapter ("Level 1: Cultural-Level Interventions"), we will offer a range of cultural-level advocacy interventions aimed at raising the visibility of sexual assault and gradually changing the broad parameters that shape the endemic sexual assault crisis.

Now consider the following four clinical-level cases:

Lisa[1] is a 34-year-old woman from Appalachia who is married with a 9-year-old daughter. Lisa called the practitioner after her handgun jammed when she tried to shoot herself in the head. She felt she just could not make things right for her husband and daughter. Several years earlier, Lisa had left her husband, a minister, after he had repeatedly raped her, as he said was his marital right

---

[1]All case examples are based on real clients, whose identities have been disguised to maintain confidentiality.

in the eyes of the church. She had lived with a crack cocaine dealer in another state for a while. After seeing her reflection in a store window, she decided to return to her husband and daughter and get off crack. Her husband took her back but raped her repeatedly and then demanded she pray to repent for her sins. Recently, her brother and then her best friend each died by suicide. Lisa feels so alone. She sees no way out of her situation. It seems it is all her fault.

Sarah is a 19-year-old Asian American woman who grew up in Boston. She was sexually molested at 13 by an older boy; she went to therapy but did not feel it helped. She decided to go farther from home to college in Kentucky, where she made good friends and joined a sorority. One evening during a party at a fraternity house, a member of the fraternity trapped her in his room, assaulted her sexually, and choked her for over an hour as the loud party continued outside his door. Sarah told her friends, but they just said that happens sometimes and she should be more careful in the future. After Sarah left college and returned to Boston, she pressed charges. However, the police were unsympathetic, and a grand jury refused to indict the rapist. Since then, Sarah has not returned to college. She feels isolated and depressed, and she cannot stop recalling the rape at times during the day and also in her dreams.

James is a 19-year-old Black college student. After drinking and partying one night while on vacation with friends, he ended up sleeping in a sleeping bag on the floor in a bedroom of the vacation home with another guy he had just met. As James tells it, they had all been drinking, and James knows he was being kind of loud and stupid. The other guy repeatedly told him to shut up, but James continued to be loud and laugh. Suddenly, the other guy jumped on James's back and shoved his face into the carpet so he could not shout or even breathe. He pulled James's pants down and shoved his fingers into James's anus, asking if he liked that and saying maybe James would shut up when he was told. The guy then slapped James on the back of the head. They both got in their sleeping bags and went to sleep. James felt he could not tell anyone. He has had recurrent flashbacks about the incident, has wondered why he did not fight back, and has puzzled about his manhood since then.

Margret is an 82-year-old widowed White woman who has had numerous health problems that make it harder for her to care for herself at home. Until recently, she had been taking several pain and sleeping medications and mainly remained in bed while recuperating from her most recent health chal-lenge. Home health care providers were stopping by to ensure Margret had her meals and took her medications. The other day, when Margret woke up, all the signs were present that someone had sexually assaulted or molested her while she was in a deep sleep due to her medication. Margret did not want to make her family or the health care agency aware of the incident because she was somewhat unsure about what had happened and she felt it was simply mortifying to talk about. Since then, she has remained on guard, startles at the least sound, sleeps poorly because she is refusing her medications, and simply cannot get the idea of the assault out of her mind.

Each of these four cases represents the endemic crisis of sexual assault but in different contexts. We will return to these cases later in this chapter ("Level 2: Clinical-Level Interventions"). After we discuss the convergence among evidence-based clinical models for treating sexual assault, we will track all four cases through the six phases of the process of change model to show how each client was turned out of their solution-generated vicious cycles and toward new investments in their goals and values.

In this chapter, we will first consider the context of sexual assault, including definitions, incidence, and other related elements. Then we will review both cultural-level and the individual clinical level of intervention. Finally, we will apply the process of change model to the cases of Lisa, Sarah, James, and Margret at the clinical intervention level.

THE CONTEXT OF SEXUAL ASSAULT: RAPE AS AN ENDEMIC CRISIS

The news reports and cases that opened this chapter are examples of the dominant influence of language and cultural context on the nature of common practice, what is considered a crisis, and what is or is not done about it. Recall once again our process of change working diagram of the therapy contract (Figure 4.2), which represents three spheres: the cultural context, the client (along with significant others), and the therapist (or practitioner or helper). In Chapter 8 on intimate partner violence, we discussed the power of the patriarchy that implicitly and explicitly invests privilege, power, and control in men and not women. (This is not to say that men cannot be assaulted or raped, because many often are. The majority of sexual assaults, however, happen to women, as we will soon discuss.) As with intimate partner violence, the major factor involved in sexual assault is the influence of privilege, power, and control, with emotional, physical, and sexual violence typically originating from those with more power and being perpetrated against those with less power. The related concept is that of control, with perpetrators taking power and choice away from those they manipulate, control, and assault against their will. Overall, sexual assault again falls in the category of an endemic crisis (as opposed to a developmental or incidental crisis, as discussed in Part I of this volume). It has been compellingly argued that rape and sexual assault are products of the overriding cultural context that privileges perpetrators.

Attractors and Tipping Points

In Chapter 2, we discussed the influence of the *attractor*, which draws all involved in a social system into a characteristic vortex that comes to represent the commonly described patterns of each given crisis. The sexual assaults described in the incidents and cases that opened this chapter are shaped by and follow similar patterns. The perpetrators have power, control, and influence. The victims/survivors are dominated and then silenced within the same context, because they fear being further harmed by shame and blame and are often not believed or are blamed for the assault. Later in this chapter, we will discuss the sexual assault cases of Lisa, Sarah, James, and Margret. Each of these cases will demonstrate how endemic rape is to society, as they show how sexual assaults are often normalized as in the case of Sarah, and make survivors feel extreme shame as in the cases of Lisa, James, and Margret.

Recall that such endemic crisis patterns require a difference that makes a difference to initiate change. That difference essentially goes against the flow of the dominant process and many times is experienced as counterintuitive. Recall as well that the difference or pattern shift need not be large or monumental (as in the fall of the Berlin Wall noted in the Introduction, this volume); rather, it may be initiated by a seemingly small kick point (or trigger) at a fortuitous point in time. At times, that slight shift can start what we might call a *virtuous cycle* that initiates amplifying change in the broader context of culture and subsequently in people's lives. Ullman (2023) suggested that the "emergence of the #MeToo movement has revealed how endemic rape is to society and has heightened awareness of the collective action of speaking out and taking action necessary to combat sexual violence including harassment, stalking, rape, and partner abuse" (p. 43). Before we discuss that movement and other cultural-level interventions, it is important to look at how sexual assault has been defined and to learn about its scope and extent.

Definitions

There are many legal and mental health–based definitions of sexual assault and rape, and they may vary by state and nation. One of the most concise definitions was offered by Ullman (2023), following that of Koss et al. (2007):

> *Rape* refers to attempted or completed forced sexual penetration or penetration obtained when a person does not or cannot consent (e.g., as a result of substance use). *Sexual assault* refers to less severe forms of sexual victimization, including unwanted sexual contact (e.g., fondling) and sexual coercion (e.g., manipulation). (p. 8, italics in the original)

Before we proceed, a note is needed on the use of the terms *victims* and *survivors* in this chapter. Following more recent literature, we will use *victim* to affirm the impact of assault and *survivor* as a term of empowerment denoting resilience in overcoming and moving beyond the assault (cf. Koss et al., 2017; Ullman, 2023).

Incidence

A study of responses to the 2016–2017 U.S. Centers for Disease Control and Prevention National Intimate Partner and Sexual Violence Survey (NISVS) indicated that one in five women reported experiencing completed or attempted rape during their lifetime, 43.6% of women (nearly 52.2 million) experienced some form of contact sexual violence in their lifetime, and 37.0% (approximately 44.3 million women) reported unwanted sexual contact (e.g., groping) in their lifetime (Basile et al., 2022). Of the victims of rape and sexual assault, 91% were female and 9% were male. In approximately 8 out of 10 cases of rape, the victim knew the person who raped them (Basile et al., 2022).

Vast Underreporting

The NISVS statistics reported by Basile et al. (2022) are certainly concerning but likely do not reflect the actual incidence of rape and sexual assault, given that there is a great reluctance to disclose—much less report—these crimes. In her excellent recent book on sexual assault, Ullman (2023, pp. 55–70) offers an overview of why, how often, and to whom women disclose, indicating that rape is one of the most underreported crimes, with 63% of sexual assaults not reported to police. Rates of disclosure to informal sources were somewhat higher, with more than half of rape survivors telling friends, a third telling family, and less than a quarter (16%) telling partners. More than 90% of sexual assault victims on college campuses do not report the assault. With this in mind, practitioners are unlikely to encounter sexual assault victims, even if they colocate with emergency rooms (ERs) or collaborate with rape crisis centers. For example, Ullman (2023) discussed the fact that rape crisis centers are still among the most rarely contacted formal resources, with only 5% to 10% of rape victims reporting using such centers.

This brings us back to the role of cultural context in our process of change working diagram (Figure 4.2). This diagram may be the best vehicle for our discussion of rape and sexual assault, including answers to the questions of why victims (or survivors) do not disclose and what efforts have been mounted at the cultural context level and the client–therapist or individual level to enhance successful access, decrease secondary victimization, and promote resolution for those who seek help. A prime example of secondary victimization comes from a set of structured interviews with 21 sexual assault survivors in Canada, following problematic contact when reporting sexual assault to police (Murphy-Oikonen et al., 2022). In summarizing their findings, Murphy-Oikonen et al. stated the following:

> The women in this study who experienced a sexual assault and reported the assault to police were hopeful that police would help them, and justice would be served. Instead, these women were faced with insensitivity, blaming questions, lack of investigation, and lack of follow-up from the police, all of which contributed to [their] not being believed by the institutions designed to protect them. (p. 12)

Let us turn now to barriers to reporting.

Barriers to Reporting

Rape and sexual assault are serious offenses. So why aren't they reported more often? Survivors cite several reasons. According to a recent U.S. Department of Justice report, 20% of survivors worry about retaliation (not just from the perpetrator, but from society at large), 13% said they think the police would not do anything to help, and, tragically, 8% said they did not think the rape or sexual assault was important enough to report (Kimble & Chettiar, 2018). The NISVS reported that only 3%–15% of young adults sought help from formal sources, including police, medical personnel, or counseling services (with police being the least frequently sought out, followed by medical personnel and counseling services) (Basile et al., 2022). Most of the barriers to disclosure occur in the cultural context, the first sphere of the process of change working diagram (Figure 4.2); others occur in the intersecting identities of the client sphere (e.g., class, gender, identity, race and ethnicity, substance use, and relation to the perpetrator). Survivors of assault with intersecting identities with less stature, power, and credibility in a given culture are among those who are least likely to disclose sexual assault. Furthermore, when the assault occurs with alcohol or drug use or when it is viewed as happening in a dating or committed marital or other relationship, survivors are also much less likely to choose to identify the assault as rape, disclose it, or take any action on it. As discussed in Chapter 8 on intimate partner violence, the most dominant contextual force driving rape and sexual assault is the patriarchy, which invests more power and control in perpetrators when they are male. Remember that power and control differences also reside in same-sex partnerships and may also involve women as perpetrators. (Interested readers should refer to Sarah Ullman's recently revised book, *Talking About Sexual Assault: Society's Response to Survivors* (2023), for a more thorough review and discussion of the contextual barriers impeding disclosure around sexual assault.) Another issue is the cultural sexualization and objectification of women through media and, more recently, through ready internet access to pornography. Although there is a vast literature on this topic, the essence of this impact is that assaults and coercions always emanate from control of those with more power exerted over those more vulnerable. With power as it relates to cultural context in mind, we now turn to cultural-level interventions that have attempted to reshape these influences on the endemic crisis of sexual assault.

LEVEL 1: CULTURAL-LEVEL INTERVENTIONS

Referring again to the three spheres of our process of change working diagram (Figure 4.2), remember that the cultural and language context of each social system shapes and guides the flow of the system (just like the banks and riverbed of Heraclitus's river discussed in Chapter 2, this volume). Therefore, shifts in cultural context relating to rape and sexual assault hold promise of shifting how these crimes are defined and responded to, how victims are supported, and how perpetrators are sanctioned. Although there have been several major attempts to shape this shift, none have been so important in the United States as the evolution of rape crisis centers in their various forms, the Violence Against Women Act (VAWA), the #MeToo movement, and the evolution of Sexual Assault Nurse Examiners (SANE nurses) in medical ERs. This section will address each of these in turn.

Rape Crisis Centers

The advent of rape crisis centers traces its history to the consciousness-raising movement on women's issues from the mid-1950s to the mid-1970s. Ullman (2023) described it as a product of what she termed *second-wave feminism*. *First-wave feminism* refers to feminist activities of the nineteenth and twentieth centuries in the United States and the United Kingdom, culminating in women's right to vote in 1920 with the Nineteenth Amendment to the U.S. Constitution. The second wave had a major element of *radical feminism*, emphasizing the social dominance of women by men across the culture and raising consciousness that social context was a major influence on crimes such as domestic violence and sexual assault. (Third- and fourth-wave feminist influences will be discussed later as they apply to more recent influences addressing intersecting identities of women and the #MeToo movement.)

In the 1970s, rape crisis centers evolved from the feminist movement positions that violence against women is a product of social control and that women can help one another transform from victim to survivor (with the use of the term *survivor* being an important shift in the influence of language within culture made in an attempt to empower women). Many of the first rape crisis centers evolved from grassroots efforts of women involved in the feminist movement, with untrained volunteers often running centers out of women's homes with donated time and materials. These egalitarian, horizontally organized groups aimed not only to offer support and advocacy for survivors but also to create social change in a patriarchal culture. Support groups were organized and run within these centers to offer women validation of their stories and the ability to share them with others in affirming environments to put blame on a misogynistic culture and reverse common feelings of guilt, shame, and self-blame typically felt by survivors. This approach offered clear *reversals* of typical rape crisis patterns.

The structure of rape crisis centers in the 1980s evolved from the early centers targeting major social changes and organizing marches (e.g., Take Back the Night, discussed later in this section) to later centers focusing on moving to service delivery, affiliating with other agencies, and taking political action (Gornick et al., 1985). Today, there are more than 1,200 rape crisis centers in the United States, with most having moved to competing for funding from government and United Way resources; these funders typically require more licensed professional staff and boards (McMahon, 2019). The most common constellation of services includes 24-hour hotlines with volunteer staff and community referrals and links, group and individual counseling and support groups, and legal and medical advocacy with volunteers and staff accompanying women through reporting, medical care, and the legal system. Many services today have become part of city and county prosecutor offices as essentially victim-witness divisions.

Violence Against Women Act of 1994

The VAWA was passed in 1994, and provided $1.6 billion toward investigation and prosecution of violent crimes against women, imposed automatic and mandatory restitution on those convicted, and allowed civil redress when prosecutors chose to not prosecute cases (Violence Against Women Act, 1994). The act also established the Office on Violence Against Women within the U.S. Department of Justice. One of the greatest successes of the VAWA is its emphasis on a coordinated community response to domestic violence, dating violence, sexual assault, and stalking. Courts, law enforcement, prosecutors, victim services, and the private bar were directed to work together in a coordinated effort that did not exist at the state and local levels.

In 2005, reauthorization of the VAWA defined what population benefited under the term *underserved populations*, described as follows:

> populations underserved because of geographic location, underserved racial and ethnic populations, populations underserved because of special needs (such as language barriers, disabilities, alien status, or age) and any other population determined to be underserved by the Attorney General or by the Secretary of Health and Human Services as appropriate. (Violence Against Women Act, 2005)

The reauthorization also amended the Omnibus Crime Control and Safe Streets Act of 1968 to "prohibit officials from requiring sex offense victims to submit to a polygraph examination as a condition for proceeding with an investigation or prosecution of a sex offense" (Violence Against Women Act, 2005).

Culture Wars and the VAWA

The monumental cultural intervention in the United States to shift positions on sexual assault and violence against women has not been without pushback from conservative sources as part of what is referred to as the *culture wars movement*. The VAWA expired in 2011, and the law was up for reauthorization in Congress in 2012. Contention arose around proposals that favored reducing services to undocumented immigrants and LGBT individuals and giving Native American tribal authorities jurisdiction over sex crimes involving non-Native American individuals on tribal lands, temporarily ending VAWA coverage after 18 years. After 2 more years of legislative fighting, the revised, stripped-down VAWA was finally passed in 2013. It allowed only limited protection for LGBT and Native American individuals but did expand federal protections to gay, lesbian, transgender, and Native American individuals as well as immigrants and victims of human trafficking (Violence Against Women Act, 2013). As evidence of the deeply entrenched views on violence against women, the VAWA has been the subject of regular disputes and threats of funding cuts or ending funding. In March 2022, it was again signed into law as part of the Consolidated Appropriations Act of 2022 (Violence Against Women Act Reauthorization Act, 2022). The 2022 VAWA reauthorization does not include provisions to cover assaults by boyfriends, owing to opposition by conservative factions.

Impressively, however, the 2022 reauthorized VAWA supports the work of community-based organizations engaged in efforts to end domestic violence, dating violence, sexual assault, and stalking, particularly those groups that provide culturally and linguistically specific services. Additionally, the 2022 reauthorized VAWA provides specific support for work with tribes and tribal organizations to end domestic violence, dating violence, sexual assault, and stalking against Native American women. The act also created the National Resource Center on Cybercrimes Against Individuals; increased support for the Rape Prevention and Education Program and for sexual assault services programs; expanded prevention education for students in higher education institutions; promoted the use of trauma-informed, victim-centered training for law enforcement personnel; and enhanced training for sexual assault forensic examiners. The reauthorized VAWA also increased funding for domestic violence and sexual assault services; reformed the military justice system to address sexual assault, harassment, and related crimes; increased resources for survivors of crime, including gender-based violence; and strengthened regional leadership on violence against Indigenous women and girls. All of these changes are an amazing and powerful reversal of the traditional context of patriarchal dominance in U.S. culture. Yet as we have discussed, these changes have gone strongly against the former current, with strong conservative pushback all the way.

International Women's Day and Take Back the Night

On a broader level, ongoing movements continue to raise the issues of inequality of women in male-dominated culture, with gradual results. International Women's Day (IWD) is held annually on March 8 to honor the achievements of women and promote women's rights (International Women's Day, 2024). IWD grew out of efforts in the early twentieth century to promote women's rights, especially suffrage. Aided by the growth of feminism in the 1960s and United Nations sponsorship in 1975, IWD experienced a revitalization in the late twentieth century. Today, it is an important occasion for promoting women's issues and rights, especially in developing countries. Take Back the Night marches are a related effort to raise cultural consciousness of patriarchal issues and bring attention to issues of safety in public places for women and girls (Take Back the Night Foundation, 2023). These marches are global grassroot community efforts that began in the 1970s. They take a variety of forms depending on local priorities, yet they typically evolve around women literally marching in the night with banners and chanting slogans about the right to walk freely and safely, and they often include emotionally charged "speak-outs" by survivors. These dovetailing movements continue to make headway in shifting the cultural context of what some have called a rape culture fueled by male-dominant norms, with some success. The U.S. Federal Bureau of Investigation (2023) reported a slight decrease in 2022 in forcible rapes compared with 1990. Yet we need to remember that rape is one of the most underreported crimes, and rape crisis centers are one of the least used resources by rape survivors (Ullman, 2023).

Returning to disclosure as a time-limited window of opportunity, conclusions from a systematic review of early interventions to sexual assault stated that "the first month post-assault is a time of increased opportunity for intervention, both because of the increased availability of formal responders during this time . . . and the higher likelihood if informal disclosure soon after the assault" (Dworkin & Schumacher, 2018, p. 461). The authors concluded by suggesting the following:

> While many effects were short-lived, interventions that were perceived positively may be associated with lower posttraumatic stress up to a year post-assault. These findings support the importance of offering best-practice interventions that are perceived positively, rather than simply encouraging survivors to seek help. (p. 459)

#MeToo Movement

Tarana Burke is an American activist from New York City, and she started the #MeToo movement. In 2006, Burke began using the hashtag #MeToo on social media to help other women with similar experiences to stand up for themselves. Over a decade later, on October 15, 2017, #MeToo went viral after the Harvey Weinstein sexual assault allegations were exposed when a tweet by Alyssa Milano encouraged people who had been sexually harassed or assaulted to write "#MeToo" on social media. The movement quickly spread internationally and in essence initiated broader acknowledgment of the extent of sexual violence through the less threatening and somewhat more anonymous medium of social media. The eventual positive feedback spiral, or virtuous cycle, can be seen in the *Time Magazine* 2017 Person of the Year, awarded to "The Silence Breakers" and featuring the faces and stories of five women on the cover who came forward publicly with their stories of sexual assault (Zacharek et al., 2017).

The impact of the #MeToo movement can be seen in the news reports we described earlier. For example, Harvey Weinstein was eventually convicted of multiple sexual assaults in New York and California with respective jail sentences of 23 and 16 years (Reuters, 2024). Weinstein's conviction in New York was overturned on the technicality that women unrelated to the case also testified. It is being relitigated as of this writing.

E. Jean Carroll's case against former President Donald Trump was a broader result of the same movement; eventually, Carroll built up the courage to write about it. In reaction, Trump punched back with a range of insulting and defamatory responses. In response, Carroll brought a defamation case against

Trump, won, and was awarded $83 million (Schonfeld, 2024). The case was being appealed as of this writing. However, it serves as a cautionary tale: although Carroll won the civil trial and was awarded damages acknowledging the impact of the prior sexual assault, Trump is the Republican nominee for the 2024 U.S. presidential election at the time of this writing.

General cultural attitudes and acceptance of sexual assault change slowly, particularly as it relates to powerful perpetrators. The Brock Turner case described earlier is yet another example, with the influence of power and privilege of a wealthy, popular elite college athlete, the vicious cross-examination of the woman assaulted, the light sentence imposed, and the eventual reempowerment of the survivor, Chanel Miller (Gersen, 2023). Miller (2020) published her experiences of the assault, the trial, and her path to survivorship in the book, *Know My Name: A Memoir*, thus retaking control of her life and story and sharing it with others. Each of the cases just discussed is a microcosm of the crisis attractor of sexual assault in a cultural context as well as the vicious and virtuous cycles around the tipping points of assault and disclosure.

Returning to the impact of the #MeToo movement, a very sophisticated recent analysis, titled "The Effects of Social Movements: Evidence from #MeToo" (Levy & Mattsson, 2023), supported the cultural impact of the #MeToo movement. Across cultures, the movement increased reporting of sex crimes by 10% during the first 6 months and persisted more than a year after it started, as individuals perceived sexual misconduct to be a more serious problem. In the year after the movement began, the average Google search interest in sexual misconduct increased by an unprecedented 85%. However, the authors stated that "the MeToo movement did not lead to major immediate changes in laws [and] [w]e do not find evidence that stigma decreased, nor do we find evidence that victims' expectations on how authorities would respond to a report changed following the movement" (pp. 3–4). Thus, although the efforts to raise the cultural visibility of sexual assault are both highly valuable and impactful, their impact in changing the endemic embedded nature of sexual assault within the cultural context moves slowly. From our discussion of chaos and catastrophe theory in Chapter 2 (this volume), it is important to recall that such slow movement often pushes systems to what has been described as a cliff or cusp where rapid, all-or-nothing shifts often occur. Only time will tell.

Sexual Assault Nurse Examiners

We now turn our focus to efforts to reshape the impact of reporting sexual assault and decrease the potential of secondary victimization, particularly in ERs and related forensic examinations. *Secondary victimization* occurs when the victim suffers further harm not as a direct result of the criminal act but due to the manner in which institutions and other individuals deal with the victim. Campbell (2005) found that as a result of their contact with ER physicians and nurses, most rape survivors stated that they felt bad about themselves (81%), guilty (74%), depressed (88%), nervous or anxious (91%), violated (94%), distrustful of others (74%), and reluctant to seek further help (80%). P. Y. Martin (2013) said that although most rape victims may have minimal physical injuries, they are sent to the ER mainly for forensic evidence collection. However, most ER physicians are triaged to more urgent emergency cases, resulting in average wait times ranging from 4 to 10 hours before examination. Furthermore, most ER physicians are not practiced in and are more reluctant to collect rape examination kits out of concern for being called into court for testimony and cross-examination. It is not uncommon, for example, for hospital ER staff to question victims about their prior sexual histories, what they were wearing at the time of the assault, what they did to "cause" the assault, why they were with the assailant in the first place (if they knew the rapist), and why they trusted the assailant (if they knew the rapist). All of this, of course, feeds back into the earlier-noted survivor responses of feeling bad about themselves, blamed, guilty, and reluctant to seek further help.

Another distressing finding regarding ER practices is that historically, often fewer than half of rape victims treated in hospital ERs receive basic services, such as emergency contraception to prevent pregnancy and information about the risk of pregnancy, sexually transmitted diseases, and HIV (Campbell, 2005). At the heart of the process view of crisis intervention is using the window of opportunity at the point of disclosure and intervention to initiate a tipping point to transform an assault victim into an empowered survivor. A major move into that window of opportunity has been the development of SANE programs.

The initial movement toward SANE programs began in the late 1970s, in metropolitan areas such as Memphis, Tennessee; Minneapolis, Minnesota; and Amarillo, Texas (Office for Victims of Crime, 2024). Over the decades, the SANE approach and its structures and training have spread throughout the United States and Canada; as of 2013, there were nearly 450 programs throughout the United States. Training typically consists of approximately 40 hours of classroom training and 40–96 hours of clinical training in evidence collection, chain-of-evidence requirements, expert testimony, injury detection and treatment, pregnancy screening, sexually transmitted disease screening and treatment, and crisis intervention around common emotional response patterns. Awareness of common response patterns is offered to normalize and predict future responses for survivors. To address survivors' psychological needs, SANEs strive to preserve victims' dignity, ensure that they are not retraumatized by the examination, and assist them in regaining control by letting them make decisions throughout the evidence collection process. Many SANE programs work with their local rape crisis centers so rape victim advocates can also be present for the examination to provide emotional support and allow nurses to eventually serve as expert witnesses in court, while the rape crisis center volunteer can offer support and advocacy from the ER through the potential courtroom proceedings.

Turning to the effectiveness of SANE programs, a smaller semistructured interview of survivors who went through a SANE experience in Canada reported that they felt respected, safe, in control, believed and supported, cared for by people with expertise, informed, and cared for beyond the hospital because they received the option for follow-up care (Ericksen et al., 2002). In an excellent comprehensive review, Campbell et al. (2005) reviewed the empirical literature regarding the effectiveness of SANE programs in five domains: psychological recovery, comprehensive medical care, accurate collection and documentation of forensic evidence, improving prosecution, and creating community change. Campbell et al. found that preliminary evidence suggested that SANE programs were effective in all domains. Furthermore, a later follow-up study compared pre-to-post outcomes of SANE across six programs representing rural, midsize, and urban areas, and the investigators found an overall significant increase in prosecutions from pre- to post-SANE time periods (Campbell et al., 2014).

However, recall the problems recounted in Chapter 4 when Western intervenors tried to impose what they felt were evidence-based approaches to dealing with trauma on the population of Sri Lanka following a devastating tsunami. That intervention likely caused more problems than it attempted to treat. A similar result was noted when the SANE nurse program was imported to Afghanistan (Zupancic et al., 2016). Researchers found that two out of three victims said other health problems were higher priority, 45% were offended by screening, and 57% were surprised that their victimization was subject to mandatory police report (Zupancic et al., 2016). The methods conflicted with cultural beliefs that these problems were better treated by home remedies and religion. This is one more reminder for those in dominant Western cultures to attend closely to the language, values, traditions, and norms of other cultures before implementing wholesale approaches found effective in their own contexts and cultures.

The Uphill Battle to Change the Cultural Context Sphere

As just described, there have been outstanding and commendable sociocultural and programmatic efforts to draw attention to sexual assault issues and to change the cultural contexts that tacitly look the other way and even perpetuate victim blaming. Yet there is clearly a long way to go. Efforts to change the cultural context are discussed next.

Bystander Intervention

On a positive note regarding reshaping attitudes and potentially interceding in future sexual assaults, work is being done to train bystanders. Recall the case of Brock Turner at the beginning of this chapter. The assault occurred on a college campus where the incidence of sexual assault ranges from 20% to 25%. Recall also that two male graduate students stepped in to stop the assault and engage police. There is longstanding research around the *bystander effect*, wherein the classic finding is reluctance to step in to stop an attack. However, more recent programs have targeted training of college students in general and sorority and fraternity members in particular in dispelling rape myths, identifying incidents of potential sexual assault, and educating on how to respond and intervene. In a systematic review of bystander interventions, Mujal et al. (2021) concluded that two programs, Bringing in the Bystander and The Men's Program, have the most consistent reliable and valid positive outcomes and share some teaching methods, which include self-efficacy through role-playing exercises and using presentation, discussion, and active learning exercises. Although these two programs are founded on different theories and present different scenarios, both use trauma-informed and evidence-based research, focus on empathy building and support for survivors and victims of sexual assault, and emphasize perceived self-efficacy, training or peer facilitation, and bystander and community importance in prevention and recovery.

Fischer et al. (2011) conducted a meta-analytic review on bystander intervention in dangerous and nondangerous emergencies. They concluded that dangerous emergencies produced smaller bystander effects than did nondangerous emergencies. For example, they found that (a) dangerous emergencies are more clearly perceived as actual emergencies; (b) additional bystanders reduce fear because they signal the possibility of social, physical, or psychological support when the focal individual contemplates intervention; and (c) dangerous emergencies are most effectively resolved by coordination and cooperation among a greater number of bystanders. Some of the greatest effects of such bystander training have thus been to help students clearly define potential sexual assault as a true emergency, to be able to identify instances as crises calling for their action, and to feel that their friends support their choice to intervene. Once more, viewing crises through a process-based lens and intervening with *all parts* of the system drives home the impact of a process view of rape and sexual assault.

Evolution of Rape Crisis Centers in Their Various Forms

Finally, an ongoing and potent element in helping to reshape the cultural sphere that perpetuates sexual assault is the Rape, Abuse & Incest National Network (RAINN). As the largest online resource repository and source of information in the United States, RAINN is a nonprofit anti–sexual-assault organization, operates the National Sexual Assault Hotline as well as the Department of Defense Safe Helpline, and carries out programs to prevent sexual assault, help survivors, and ensure that perpetrators are brought to justice through victim services, public education, public policy, and consulting services (Rape, Abuse & Incest National Network, 2024b). The RAINN toll-free hotline is available 24 hours a day, 7 days a week and routes callers to the nearest sexual assault service provider; it received its one-millionth caller as of 2006. RAINN continues to be one of the most influential forces for ongoing changes in laws and providing support and resources for rape survivors. The organization's website (https://www.rainn.org/) is a testament to its efforts to help survivors, educate the public, improve public policy, and consult and train. However, RAINN has not avoided the ongoing culture wars or the polemic debate around bringing perpetrators to justice versus changing cultural norms and values that breed sexual violence. Evidence of that debate can be seen in two 2014 *Time Magazine* editorials, titled "It's Time to End 'Rape Culture' Hysteria" (Kitchens, 2014) and its rejoinder "Rape Culture Is Real" (Maxwell, 2014), and the consequent viral hashtag, #RapeCultureIsWhen. Historically, there has always been pushback from conservative positions on issues surrounding sexual assault, as we discussed in the battles around the VAWA discussed earlier. However, the truth always lies in the middle as a "both-and" position. In fact, RAINN has advocated for a three-pronged approach for combating rape: empowering community members through bystander intervention education, as reviewed earlier, using "risk-reduction messaging" to encourage students to increase their personal safety, and promoting clearer education on "where the 'consent line' is" (Rape, Abuse & Incest National Network, 2024b). RAINN also offers a range of resources for survivors and intervenors, which we will take up in the subsequent discussion of rape trauma syndrome (RTS) within the client and practitioner spheres of our process of change working diagram (Figure 4.2) for individuals who come forward seeking help in recovering from sexual assault.

LEVEL 2: DIRECT CLINICAL INTERVENTIONS

Practitioners need to be aware of the ongoing efforts to shift the cultural context, as reviewed in the previous section. These efforts are slowly shifting the cultural elements that underlie the perpetuation of sexual assault and the barriers to victims considering disclosing, much less following through with, reporting, examinations, and prosecution without encountering secondary victimization at the hands of those designated as helpers.

However, there is a range of knowledge and practices available to help individuals who come to the attention of practitioners to find resolution and even resilience and growth following an assault. A set of important elements of the process of change perspective related to intervention include being aware of any generic patterns or solution-generated problems around each crisis, and then remaining open to all unique or specific variations. Then the main interventions revolve around understanding the values, goals, language, and culture that shape the survivor's attempts to deal with the aftermath of the sexual assault. The final steps are to track the vicious cycles around the individual's situation, design interventions to interdict and reverse those patterns, and then support the pattern shifts once they begin. First, we will address RTS as a potential generic pattern, then we will review the critiques of that concept and offer a general overview of successful evidence-supported interventions available for rape and sexual assault. Finally, we will track how those interventions align with the general process of change perspective as it weaves its way through this pressing crisis.

Rape Trauma Syndrome as a Potential Generic Pattern

RTS was first identified as a generic response pattern by Burgess and Holmstrom (1974). This syndrome has been described as a cluster of psychological and physical signs, symptoms, and reactions common to most rape victims immediately following a rape, but which can also occur for months or years afterward. As noted earlier, RAINN offers information on RTS as a resource for survivors, with tools to help them understand, normalize, and potentially negotiate the aftermath of sexual assault. RTS is commonly described as moving through three phases (Rape, Abuse & Incest National Network, 2024a): The *acute phase* occurs immediately after the assault and lasts from a few days to several weeks. Reactions are said to fall into three categories: (a) expressed open emotion, (b) flat affect bordering on shock, and (c) shocked disbelief and disorientation. The acute phase is followed by an *outward adjustment phase*, which includes coping mechanisms such as (a) minimization, suggesting things could have been worse; (b) obsessive thinking about the assault; (c) refusals to discuss the assault; (d) consistent analysis of why the assault happened; or (e) flight, including moving and changing jobs, appearance, or relationships. Finally, in the *resolution phase*, the assault is no longer the central focus of the individual's life. Often the individual will begin to accept the rape as part of their life and choose to move on. To its credit, this generic model has evolved and now assumes that individuals will take steps forward and backward and that, although there are phases, it is not a linear progression and will be different for every person. This model of RTS has been used for years to train practitioners in how to anticipate and guide their work with survivors, and it has some overall merit in normalizing survivors' reactions to assaults and inoculating assault survivors against overreacting to some of the phases as they move forward.

Critiques of RTS

The RTS model has been subject to some extensive critiques in recent years. Given that most sexual assaults are committed by someone the survivor knows, many assaults involve less force and include varied situations; thus, most survivors are more likely to experience more self-blame and guilt, which modifies the RTS picture. Furthermore, many have criticized the description of the response patterns as a "syndrome," thus pathologizing survivors' behaviors, which are better viewed as reasonable reactions to unreasonable and distressing contexts. In a thorough review of the literature, O'Donohue et al. (2014) presented the following conclusions on RTS: it is vague in important details; it is unclear what its boundary conditions are; it uses unclear terms that do not have a basis in psychological science; it fails to specify key quantitative relationships; it has not undergone subsequent scientific evaluation since the Burgess and Holmstrom (1974) study; there are theoretical allegiance effects; it has not achieved a consensus in the field; it is not falsifiable; it ignores possible mediators; it is not culturally sensitive; and it is not suitable for being used to infer that rape has or has not occurred. Consensus has arisen that a preferable description of general responses to sexual assault is better referred to in terms of posttraumatic stress disorder (PTSD), discussed in Chapter 5 of this volume.

Recalling many of the critiques of the PTSD diagnosis from Chapter 5, a comprehensive review of the harm done by rape (Wasco, 2003) summarizes the literature by saying that "the diagnostic classification of posttraumatic stress disorder (PTSD), when used as a lens for viewing sexual violence, may restrict our understanding of survivors' experiences" (p. 309). Wasco (2003) advocated for a more contextual understanding and further noted that "A recent review of ethnocultural research suggests that although intrusive thoughts and memories of the traumatic event may be commonly experienced in many cultural groups, symptoms of avoidance/numbing and hyperarousal may differ according to one's ethnocultural affiliation" (p. 314). Furthermore, far from violating a victim's belief that a rape has shattered their sense of a just world, Wasco reminded us, "For some victims, rape may confirm assumptions that violence is a routine part of life or that they do not have sexual control over their bodies" (p. 313). Ecological models may better account for varying reactions to rape. To this end, Koss et al. (2017) advocated for an emphasis on "victim voice" in reenvisioning responses to sexual and physical violence nationally and internationally. Turning to the therapist or practitioner sphere of our three-sphere process of change working diagram (Figure 4.2), Koss et al. emphasized (a) *cultural humility*, which they described as an expansive process of conducting self-reflection, breaking down power dynamics, and committing to a mutual and ongoing learning experience; and (b) *radical listening* through overcoming personal biases to become truly attentive to the critical issues and goals being expressed by speakers. Koss et al. advocated for "accepting answers without judgment, especially when the input is uncomfortable, challenging preconceptions of victim needs, letting go of biases toward current responses and shifting the center of power back to victims" (p. 16). This approach emphasizes locating individual and community strengths rather than focusing on deficits and rejecting the idea of a one-size-fits-all intervention as standardized views and approaches are applied to assist survivors.

Effective Interventions With Sexual Assault Survivors

Here, we explore the question of what interventions might be effective and available for practitioners to access when responding to victims of sexual assault and rape when they do disclose and seek help to move beyond their current distress. If we can agree now that there is not a "one-size-fits-all" approach, is there a set of relatively common response patterns that have been successfully identified? Is there a common thread running through them? And if there are several effective approaches, how might one choose among them?

Most Common Response Patterns

With acknowledgment of the cautions listed earlier against assuming all sexual assault and rape victims will struggle with the same problems, there is still some general agreement around the most common difficulties experienced by a majority of survivors. Again, these are what we have termed *generic crisis response patterns*, which will always be modified by specific factors of cultural and individual context. They are also the most common difficulties addressed in the major clinical approaches to treatment.

As noted earlier, many of the patterns described in response to RTS and PTSD also commonly occur after sexual assault, including flashbacks, nightmares, startle responses, hypervigilance, avoidance, self-blame, guilt, and depression, among others. In many ways, the overriding patterns of these efforts to resolve the aftermath of sexual assault cluster around efforts to *master by avoidance*; often, the more the individual tries to suppress, avoid, or put the incident out of their mind, the more it recurs seemingly spontaneously. These challenges seem to be related to survivors who have experienced secondary trauma through negative reactions from others or who have delayed or not disclosed the assault until appearing for treatment (Ahrens et al., 2010). Research reviews converge on the following conclusion offered by Kennedy and Prock (2018):

> Self-blame (general, behavioral, and characterological), shame, and negative social reactions are linked to a host of poor outcomes, including PTSD, depression, psychological and physical distress, affect dysregulation, social withdrawal, maladaptive coping and beliefs, and reduced self-esteem; [further,] longitudinal analyses indicate that self-blame, anticipatory stigma–related nondisclosure, and negative reactions predict sexual revictimization. (p. 9)

The authors also affirmed that "Survivors from a disadvantaged social location appear to report higher levels of stigmatization and stigma in comparison to their more advantaged peers" (p. 10).

The Paradox of Effective Interventions

Analyses from the process perspective of the literature across most effective psychotherapy approaches indicate that counterintuitive or paradoxical shifts and reversals of most problem patterns are at the heart of their effectiveness (Fraser, 2018; Fraser & Solovey, 2007b). These shifts and reversals are also fundamental to most approaches to crisis intervention (Fraser, 1995c, 2001). This is what we have discussed as *second-order change*, or a major change of the overriding ideas and patterns around the vicious cycles of problems.

It is not surprising, then, that all of the major approaches that research has found effective in resolving the sequelae of rape and sexual abuse involve variations of *exposure* to memories of the assault and *reframing* of the beliefs underlying self-blame and guilt. According to the literature, these approaches include prolonged exposure (PE) therapy (Foa et al., 2018; McLean & Foa, 2011), cognitive behavior therapy (CBT)–based interventions (Lomax & Meyrick, 2022), brief cognitive processing therapy (B-CPT; Nixon et al., 2016), and eye movement desensitization and reprocessing (EMDR; Covers et al., 2021), among others. Each of these approaches is based on somewhat different premises and procedures, yet each combines exposure and cognitive restructuring—both core elements of second-order change in the process of change perspective.

Broad-Based Effectiveness

Relating back to the literature examining these approaches, an earlier study (Anderson & Frank, 1991) comparing CBT, systematic desensitization, brief psychoeducation, and psychological support found significant reductions in depression and fear with *all* interventions over the 1-year follow-up, with no significant differences between groups. These findings suggest that the brief interventions were equivalent to intensive treatments. Nixon et al. (2016) demonstrated that an evidence-based trauma-focused therapy such as CPT or more traditional approaches to rape crisis counseling can be effective when delivered as an early intervention for acute stress responses to sexual assault. Finally, in a recent systemic review of the effectiveness of psychological interventions in sexual assault, Lomax and Meyrick (2022) concluded:

> Together these studies provide tentative support for the use of early CBT-based interventions in reducing or preventing posttraumatic stress, with the strongest support found for multi-session treatments involving exposure and processing of the trauma such as B-CPT and modified PE. These interventions were used with women presenting with high levels of acute distress who are also at the greatest risk of developing PTSD. (p. 322)

Miles et al. (2024) conducted a systematic review of evidence-based treatments for adolescent and adult sexual assault victims. Their findings confirmed those of the U.S. Department of Veterans Affairs and the U.S. Department of Defense clinical practice guidelines for management of PTSD and acute stress disorder, showing strong evidence for the use of PE therapy, CPT, and EMDR, among other closely related approaches. In essence, nearly all organized treatment approaches to sexual assault involve exposure and cognitive reframing, yet most are based on different basic premises underlying their approaches.

This research is just one more example of the golden thread of the process of change view weaving its way across another crisis and its interventions. When it comes to which intervention to choose, the literature recommends fitting the approach to both the views and skills of the practitioner as well as to the identities, language, and context of the survivor. Again, this reflects *flexibility* and *fit*, as described throughout this book (Fraser, 2018; Norcross, 2002). Practitioners need to flex their approaches to fit their clients. Although one size does not fit all, *all* approaches converge on the process-based premises that effective interventions almost always involve vicious cycle pattern shifts and reversals along with alterations of the ideas of clients who have shaped those patterns.

Posttraumatic Growth From Sexual Assault

It is important to remember that the process of change perspective seeks to initiate slight positive shifts, building on positives, to initiate positive feedback cycles. Remember from Chapter 5 on trauma (this volume) that there is significant literature not only on traumatic stress but also on posttraumatic growth. In their classic work, Tedeschi and Calhoun (1996) first coined the term *posttraumatic growth*, referring to the phenomenon then being noticed in the literature that a significant number of people actually experience positive outcomes following traumatic events. Their Posttraumatic Growth Inventory measures five domains, including greater appreciation of life and a changed sense of priorities; warmer, more intimate relationships with others; a greater sense of personal strength; recognition of new possibilities or paths for one's life; and spiritual development. According to Tedeschi and Calhoun (1996), "Each of the five domains of posttraumatic growth tends to have a paradoxical element to it that represents a special case of the general paradox of this field: that out of loss there is gain" (p. 6). Paradox is, of course, a hallmark of second-order change in the process of change view. Tedeschi and Calhoun concluded that many people facing trauma experience growth from their struggle. It is the process of struggle following the event that is critical to the eventual positive or negative trajectory. It becomes a potential window of opportunity. Although the traumatic event is never desirable, the good that comes out of the process of having to struggle with it is what defines potential growth. This could not be a better validation for our earlier discussion (Chapter 2 and elsewhere in this volume) of chaos theory, cusps, and essential tipping points in open social systems. It is not the nature of the trigger or the traumatic crisis point that determines the outcome; rather, it is the *context* and *process* that follows that determines future positive or negative paths.

In reviewing the literature on posttraumatic growth and sexual violence, Ulloa et al. (2016) found the same growth phenomenon in the aftermath of sexual assault. They reported a range of growth experiences in their reviewed studies:

> [Some participants reported] greater appreciation for life, whereas participants in other studies experienced growth due to their relationships with others and support from family and friends . . . others reported that the growth experienced after sexual assault was an increase in the quality and satisfaction in their relationships with their mothers as well as an increase in reported empathy for others. Spiritual change was also a theme in the articles reviewed, as were personal strength and sense of control over the situation. (p. 5)

Posttraumatic growth potential is not always found, however. The authors also stated that

> suffering sexual violence and assault more than once does seem to hinder growth. When investigating revictimization (which often occurs by a husband or family member), it has been found that growth can be severely hindered. Researchers believe that revictimization results in a perceived lack of social support, a reduction

in trust and perceived safety, and a reduced likelihood that the victim will report the assault, all of which are suspected to be key in victims' recovery. (p. 7)

Several studies suggest that as the number of symptoms increases or the severity of the PTSD and depressive symptoms increases, less growth will occur. In terms of supporting growth following sexual assault, Ulloa et al. (2016) stated the following:

> trust in an individual's support systems and spirituality have been shown to be both a predictor and consequence of growth. The limited research that looks at sexual violence victims has shown that these two aspects of a victim's life can help find positivity in trauma and counseling can further develop them to increase the possibility of growth. (p. 10)

Thus, as practitioners, it is important that we validate the impact of the assault or assaults, yet always look for strengths and support positives not only to foster resilience but also to open options for growth. In our earlier discussion of the Chinese characters for crisis, *wei jei* (Preface, this volume), we explained that the symbol for *wei* refers to danger and *jei* refers to opportunity: Remember the *jei* (opportunity), as this is more accurately related to what is done by all involved at those dangerous tipping points!

APPLYING THE PROCESS OF CHANGE MODEL

When we introduced the process of change model of how to *do* crisis intervention from the process view of crisis and crisis intervention in Chapter 4, we illustrated it by applying its key components to four cases introduced in that chapter. Because this is the last chapter of Part II, it is only fitting that we use the same format to apply the intervention model to the four cases presented at the beginning of this chapter. Next we will show how each phase of the model was applied to each of the cases in turn, starting with relationship establishment and moving on through the phases of information gathering, consensual problem formation (including goal setting, treatment rationale, and plan), break/recess, problem solving and interventions, and, finally, summary and closure. To follow the more narrative format of Chapter 4, we will start with the context of each case. Taking each example in turn, we will see the basic elements of the process of change view.

Determining the Context

To start, there is always a context and history within which each crisis occurs. Consider our four case examples.

As a 34-year-old married White Appalachian woman with a child, Lisa had lived a life of challenges and distress. She originally left her minister husband because of his regular sexual assaults. Her history of crack addiction and previous abandonment of her husband and child presented other challenges. In terms of context, this is an example of marital rape, which has only relatively recently been deemed illegal yet continues to be hard to prosecute.

As a 19-year-old Asian American college student, Sarah was bright and wanted to be independent. Leaving her close Asian family to go away to college violated their traditions in subtle ways. Sarah had two prior sexual abuse occurrences at age 13, which increased her vulnerability. The disappointment with prior therapy also presented a risk for future intervention. In terms of context, this is an example of a case of intoxication and risky choices by a survivor of assault, which has traditionally been challenging to prosecute and defend.

As a 19-year-old Black college student, James had always tried to fit into the tough athletic norms of his group of friends. The sexual assault by a man directly challenged both his view of the guys he was hanging out with and his own sense of masculinity. In terms of context, this case is an example of sexual assault of a male victim, which is rarely reported, underresearched, underresourced, and rarely prosecuted.

As a homebound 82-year-old White widow with health challenges, Margret had become reliant on home health care agents. She had always prided herself on her strength, and her current restrictions saddened her. She had been feeling increasingly isolated from friends, many of whom had already passed away, and from her family who lived farther away. In terms of context, this is a case of elder sexual assault, which is also underreported, is rarely prosecuted, and is popularly not considered to occur by the general public.

Identifying the Kick Point

All crises begin with a kick point, trigger, or perceived significant shift or difference that is viewed as dangerous and likely to threaten those involved. Consider the four cases:

- For Lisa, the kick point for her current crisis were two deaths by suicide of people close to her: her brother, who apologized for not believing or supporting her through her abuse, and her best friend, who had also been the victim of repeated sexual assault by her partners.

- For Sarah, the kick point was the violent sexual assault by a man at college. It repeated her earlier sense of vulnerability and lack of safety.

- For James, the kick point was a violent sexual assault by another guy in his group. It violated his sense of safe belonging in that group, along with his own sense of strength and masculinity.

- For Margret, the kick point was a suspected sexual assault. It not only disgusted her but also affirmed her vulnerability and validated her feeling of being alone with no help or support. It caused both embarrassment and shame.

Tracking the Solution Patterns

There is always a reaction targeting resolution of the perceived crisis by all those involved and shaped by their common life patterns, context, and history.

- Lisa had the unfortunate history of having a close relative and a close friend die by suicide. They had used guns, and Lisa had one available to use. She saw no end to the constant accusations from and repeated rapes by her husband. She felt both shame and guilt and saw killing herself as the best resolution.

- Sarah actually shared the rape at the fraternity with her sorority sisters, yet they offered no help other than telling her to be more careful. When she returned home and filed charges, she was again unsupported by the police and the courts. She felt alienated by her family who said she had risked too much when she left her home and family.

- James's major solution pattern was to shut down, not share with his friends and family, and continually downplay everything, while engaging in more sports and making risky choices.

- Margret limited all communications with her family (telling them she was fine), refused to take her medications, and fought sleep. She tried to put the incident out of her mind but it kept returning as flashbacks to what may have happened.

Identifying Potential Generic and Specific Vicious Cycles

There is an inevitable response to the solution attempts, sometimes resulting in resolution or assimilation of the perceived crisis event, yet often evolving into ongoing vicious cycles. Sometimes these vicious cycles resemble common generic patterns around the crisis according to the literature on the problem. Sometimes they are unique to the case.

- Lisa continued a cycle of self-blame and shame, while continually trying to placate her husband and care for her daughter, who blamed her for leaving. Lisa numbed herself during each repeated rape by her husband. She felt she could not share what was happening with anyone due to embarrassment.

- Sarah continued to try to push back against her abuse and abuser and share with others, only to have them deny, deflect, and often blame her for the assault both now and in the past. The more she tried, the more isolated she felt.

- James's solution pattern was to simply deny the incident, try to put it out of his mind, and overcompensate for his self-doubted masculinity. The more he continued this pattern, the more he had flashbacks and the more depressed he became.

- Margret also tried to shut down her distress by taking precautions she thought could maintain her safety, including not sharing the incident with others and trying not to be in unsafe situations in the future.

All of these cycles are variations on classic patterns of solution-generated cycles that mainly include denial and self-blame. The only variation was Sarah, who was met with common responses from others who implicitly blamed her for the assaults while isolating her.

Determining Goals

There are always goals for resolving each crisis by all involved.

- Lisa's goal was to repent and make things right for her husband, child, and family.

- Sarah's goal was to be confirmed in her victimization and supported in gaining justice.

- James's goal was to regain his former happy-go-lucky self, along with his self-respect and feeling of masculinity.

- Margret's goal was to regain her sense of safety, along with her lifelong feeling of self-assured independence.

Finding and Supporting Values and Strengths

There is always a need to accept, respect, and utilize the views, values, strengths, and resources of those involved around the perceived crisis.

- Lisa's strengths were her resiliency in the face of adversity and her caring nature for others.

- Sarah's strengths were her resilience and strength in the face of both adversity and lack of support.

- James's strengths were his striving to remain engaged in his life and with his friendships and athleticism.

- Margret's strengths were her sense of self-reliance and willingness to take on challenges.

Identifying Needed Pattern Reversals

Each crisis involves a vicious cycle to be interdicted and reversed. As practitioners identify these cycles, they can target the goals of change and the frames and rationales needed to help those reversals make sense to those involved.

- Lisa needed to step forward with her husband and child instead of withdrawing.

- Sarah needed to enlist her family for support and go toward her desired goals.

- James needed to share his situation while integrating the trauma by engaging with it.

- Margret needed to reopen with others and accept their help to regain her independence.

Matching Frames and Treatment Rationales to Fit Clients

Successful interventions always affirm the distress and embrace the goals and values of all involved as they turn the patterns around the crises to interdict and redirect vicious cycles. When evidence-supported interventions are used, they are always adapted and fit to the parties involved.

- Lisa needed to regain her strength and caring nature to make things right. Women were always the strong heart of Appalachian families.

- Sarah needed to relink with the Asian traditions of her family to gain strength and affirmation in her journey of self-discovery and ultimate fulfillment.

- James needed to acknowledge that strong males confronted adversity directly and gained strength and pride through trusting themselves and others as a team.

- Margret needed to share her adversity and distress with her family as a lesson for them, while sharing what happened with the home health care providers to make sure others would be safe in the future.

Involving and Enlisting Significant Others

The network of significant others involved around the perceived crisis always needs to be identified and their positions and responses to the crisis must be considered, because they may either contribute to the vicious cycles of the crisis or aid in its resolution.

- Lisa needed to reach out to others in her family, share her situation with them, and allow them to touch base with her therapist. She also needed to be willing to join a women's group for survivors of sexual assault and intimate partner violence for support, validation, and resources.

- Sarah needed to share the incident with her family and invite them to meet with the practitioner to discuss her situation and enlist their support to learn more about their family traditions and support her journey.

- James needed to reach out to his best friend and invite him to a meeting with the practitioner to gain his support and set out a different plan within their friendship network going forward.

- Margret first received validation from the practitioner and affirmation of her suspected sexual assault as not uncommon. She agreed to meet with the home health care agency representative along with the practitioner. She also agreed to contact her children and invite them to talk by telephone with the practitioner, who enlisted their support.

Initiating Pattern Reversals Both Within and Outside Sessions

Interventions inevitably target pattern shifts and reversals in the escalating vicious cycles. All four clients were validated in their courage and strength to share their situations with the practitioners, thus beginning a process of empowering them from the start.

- Lisa agreed to come in immediately to meet with the practitioner. She also agreed to bring in her gun and ammunition. She reached out to her sister from the practitioner's office, and her sister agreed to have Lisa stay with her. Lisa also agreed to join a women's group for survivors of sexual assault and intimate partner violence. She also contacted her husband to tell him she would be staying with her sister. She picked her daughter up from school and both stayed at her sister's house. Lisa joined the women's group while continuing to stay with her sister and daughter. She eventually filed for divorce.

- Sarah agreed to share with her family that she had sought therapy again and invited them to join the next session, where she further shared her assault and struggles to move on. In session, all discussed their Asian heritage, beliefs, and traditions and agreed to build on them. Sarah also began the process of mindfully recalling the recent sexual assault as well as those of the past, followed by reflection and a process of integrating them into who she was. Sarah eventually enrolled in a university in the Boston area, living with family at first and eventually moving out with friends. Her nightmares and flashbacks eventually receded and were experienced no more.

- James contacted his best friend and told him he had been distressed recently and sought help; James did not share the sexual assault with his best friend at that point. His friend agreed to come to a session, and James and the practitioner shared the sexual assault the way it happened. James's friend was angry at the perpetrator and shared his support for James. They agreed to both confront their acquaintance as they could. Meanwhile, the friend shared his admiration for James in sharing with him and said he would not know what to do if it had happened to him. They agreed that this was the other guy's issue, not James's. As with Sarah, James spent several more sessions with the practitioner, engaging in mindful replaying of the assault, followed by perspective taking and externalizing the issue to his perpetrator instead of himself. His flashbacks and nightmares also disappeared. James and his friend moved forward with their other friends, enjoying partying and sports as they had in the past.

- Margret agreed to call her children from the practitioner's office to share what she suspected had happened. They agreed to come for a visit to be with her and help sort things out with her physician and the home health care agency. The home health care agency thanked Margret and said they would track down the worker assigned to her care at that time and see that they were removed from employment. Margret also agreed to spend several sessions in mindful recollection of the moment when she suspected the assault, followed by discussion and support for her efforts to enlist her strength in confronting it and regaining her independence as best she could at this phase of her life. She agreed to renew taking her medications to regain her health, and she eventually agreed to move into an assisted living center with the support of her children.

Supporting Changes and Attributing Them to the Client

Once a small pattern shift begins, then it is supported, amplified, and generalized and the success is attributed to those involved rather than the practitioner. The four clients in our case examples, as well as their support networks, were congratulated for their strength in confronting the sexual assaults. The practitioners noted that such support and strength did not always happen; they asked the clients how they had all managed it and shared how they admired them for their strength.

Predicting and Prescribing Relapses to Build Resilience

Relapses ("fire drills") are predicted and prescribed before termination to build resilience. As each of these clients experienced recovery from their flashbacks and distress, they each agreed to see whether they could revisit their memories of what had happened and note their responses both within and between sessions. Although each said they had felt some understandable distress, they all felt a sense of mastery over the assault, pride in their strengths, and hope for their lives going forward.

Finishing Interventions With Congratulations and Invitations to Return

Clients are always invited to return for a "booster" visit or whenever another possible challenge occurs. The return visits are typically framed as an episode-of-care model, similar to that of family practitioners (cf. Koss & Shiang, 1994), with brief checkups as needed.

All of the clients just described were grateful for the interventions and agreed to return in the future as needed. They truly did see the practitioner as another trusted family professional resource, like their other health care providers. A few clients touched base to say how they were doing.

Once more, these cases are unique examples of interventions with sexual assault using a process perspective and the process of change model. All of the interventions included the general evidence-supported themes of validating the distress and normalizing client responses as expected given the nature of the assaults. The practitioners reframed the assaults and supported the clients' values and strengths. They fit intervention plans and rationales so they made sense to and were supported by the clients. They empowered clients in their choices, engaged those choices in the problem-generated system and networks, and, finally, supported everyone's strengths and helped them to accept changes as their own doing. Both generic patterns and unique variations were acknowledged and accommodated. All of these efforts parallel what we reviewed earlier as recommended best practices in intervention, yet it is important to remember to flex them into an intervention model that fits each unique case.

FOLLOWING THE PROCESS

In the case of sexual assault, we have found that the cultural contexts privileging perpetrators tend to breed its foundations. When survivors of assault adopt these cultural beliefs and traditions, they often blame themselves, feel guilty, and remain reluctant to disclose, much less to seek alternatives. Intervention in this endemic crisis using the process of change model addresses two levels—one of cultural change, and the other of clinical intervention—as follows:

- Creating visibility for the extent of sexual assault in the culture, enacting laws to criminalize such assaults, and building both advocacy and intervention services has gone a long way in bringing attention to the issues of sexual assault and creating options to decrease it.

- With survivors, the main interventions are to *externalize* the responsibility to the culture and the batterer and not the survivor, to *empower* the survivor by offering many choices and by admiring their strengths in the face of such adversity, to *reframe* the survivor's beliefs about the assault, to *open the system* to others if possible to decrease isolation, and to decrease traumatic stress through exposure in any ways possible.

- There are several effective exposure-oriented intervention models for survivors, similar to those for PTSD, and they are *all equally effective*. The task of the practitioner is to find an intervention that will make the most sense to the survivor and thus help make approaches such as exposure make sense.

- Finally, the practitioner should always look for strengths in the survivor and build on them. It is always possible that the most recent crisis will initiate a new direction that may produce growth.

10

TIPPING POINTS AND WINDOWS OF OPPORTUNITY

Crises are all tipping points. They represent critical points when the choices made during these time-limited windows may set a future course for either danger or opportunity. We have tracked the literature on a number of different crises and found that they invariably start with a key tipping point or trigger and then evolve into vicious cycles of repeated efforts to resolve them. The vicious cycles around the different crises tend to form generic patterns, shaped by culture and language traditions and found in the literature to be characteristic of each type of crisis. When practitioners encounter clients in crisis, they have the opportunity to meet those clients at another tipping point. Clients at these points tend to be highly motivated to change and are thus more open to influence than at any previous time during the escalating cycle of their crisis. When practitioners understand the generic patterns of the encountered crisis and the specific variations of the people and agencies involved, they can bond with and validate the pain of those involved, find a fitting rationale to explain the crisis, and then implement a typically counterintuitive shift that will create a new trigger in the lives of the clients. Once the client is triggered in this new direction, the task

https://doi.org/10.1037/0000445-011
Crisis Intervention: Using Tipping Points to Achieve Transformative Change in Therapy, by J. S. Fraser

of the practitioner is to support a new and now virtuous cycle toward *transformation* and resolution. Embracing these crisis points should become the priority of all practitioners.

Recall the Chinese characters, *wei ji*, that symbolize crisis, as we discussed in the Preface of this volume. Although it is true that *wei* symbolizes danger, *ji* is better interpreted as an incipient moment or a crucial time when something begins to change, requiring something like quick-wittedness and resourcefulness (Mair, 2009). It is how those facing these crisis points, along with those practitioners and helpers involved, view these tipping points, and what actions everyone takes, that becomes most crucial.

In this book, we traced the important history of the idea of intervening in organized ways within systems in crisis, and we noted the implicit assumptions underlying most traditional crisis approaches that adopt a homeostatic model of systems. From this view, stability is assumed to be the norm, and crises present a threat to that presumed stability. Therefore, most traditional crisis intervention has focused on reducing these risks to stability and returning the systems to their assumed precrisis stable states. This fundamental, unexamined premise has continued to draw all involved around crises and crisis intervention—including those involved in the system, such as family and friends, agencies responding to these crises, and helping professionals and practitioners—into what we have termed *solution-generated problems* and *problem-generated systems*. In essence, this risk management stance has often created vicious cycles or exacerbated existing ones. It simply has not made sense *not* to act directly to prevent or limit the danger of these situations.

The literature on the threat-rigidity cycle, the concepts of first- and second-order change, and Daniel Kahneman's (2011) Nobel Prize–winning notions of thinking fast and slow using Systems 1 and 2 all converge on the main dilemma of people in crisis. In essence, these concepts reiterate that what we have come to assume are tried-and-true notions of how things are and how to solve problems in our lives will regularly be applied over and again at crisis points, with the motto, "If at first you don't succeed—try, try again!" Changing from this typical pattern often feels dangerous and even counterintuitive or paradoxical. This frame and these efforts at crisis points initiate or exacerbate what we see across all crises as *vicious cycles*. Choices at these critical crisis points often do not resolve these crises; instead, they set those involved on a path toward further danger.

This book introduced an alternate model of open social systems, like the ones within which we all live, as a process-based perspective. Instead of viewing human interaction as stable, balanced, and resistant to change, the process level of systems emphasizes *continual change* as the basis of our lives.

Furthermore, our interactions within these process-based systems evolve or cocreate our ideas about ourselves, others, and the world within which we all live. These ideas thus help to shape the patterns of our daily lives and direct us on what to do when those ideas and presumed stable patterns are threatened. At perceived crisis points, we can either assimilate these ideas into our regular life patterns or adjust those them and our interactions going forward to adapt to the change presented by the crisis point. Failing either of these two options, we enter the common triggers or tipping points for the vicious cycles that are the basis of all crises.

We traced the history of the process-based perspective through the ancient philosophies of Heraclitus's dictum of never being able to step into the same river twice, Lao Tzu's Taoist view of balance and the watercourse way, and the more recent process philosophy of Alfred North Whitehead (1978), who reminded us that everything flows, and all is in the process of changing (see Chapter 2, this volume). Currently, research on the properties of open systems through dynamical systems theory, chaos, and catastrophe theories reiterates Leonardo da Vinci's drawings of turbulence and repeated vicious cycles, replicated in the "fractal" patterns at all levels of open systems. In such process-based systems, all involved are typically drawn into common attractors or classic vortices shaped by the constraints (in our case, our beliefs and norms) of the system. Furthermore, although change is constant, change may also be sudden and all-or-nothing and at times initiated by what appears to be a small shift or trigger. (This becomes a critical point to remember as we plan to initiate often relatively small pattern shifts in viewing or doing of all involved in a crisis point.) We need to embrace all of these principles of a process view of open social systems as we address perceived crises and as we do crisis intervention.

The process of change view reminds us that crises are not simply "out there"; rather, they are defined and acted on based on the language, norms, and individual histories of all involved. Sometimes a perceived unexpected change is simply adapted to; other times, the change initiates classic vicious cycles of failed resolution. These repeated vicious cycle patterns tend to take form and repeat themselves over and again going forward so that small samples will likely represent the crisis pattern over time. Such perceived crises may be initiated by developmental changes of the system, such as birth, death, partnering, and so on. They may also be incidental, or the product of often random events or gradually evolving tipping points that may result in thoughts or actions of suicide, among other crises. Or they may occur and reoccur as a product of elements of the cultural context, as we have tracked in the crises of intimate partner violence and sexual assault (Chapters 8 and 9, this volume). These situations may be initiated by a small tipping point shift, or they may be transformed by what often seem to be equally small yet frequently counterintuitive shifts at points when the system opens to outside input, such as from a practitioner during crisis intervention. Thus, the goal of all crisis intervention from this process of change view is simply to shift the pattern and then provide support while the seeds of that shift create new and virtuous cycles of *transformation* in the lives of all involved.

Practically speaking, we tracked doing crisis intervention through the process of change by keeping the following general set of principles in mind:

1. always attend to the context and history of the crisis;

2. look for the kick point or trigger for the crisis;

3. track the solution patterns of all involved;

4. honor the values, language, norms, traditions, and goals of all involved and align with them;

5. given the observed vicious cycle patterns, target pattern shifts and reversals;

6. accept, respect, and utilize the views, values, strengths, and resources of all involved;

7. engender a positive working relationship by affirming distress and embracing the goals and values of all involved;

8. find a frame for understanding the crisis and offer a rationale for moving forward with actions that might have formerly been counterintuitive; and

9. initiate a small yet significant shift in concepts, actions, or both to create pattern shift, and then support, amplify, and generalize the shift while attributing new positive patterns to those involved rather than to the practitioner, creating the seeds of a virtuous cycle from a vicious one.

The practical steps of the process of change model of intervention include the following:

- bonding and forming a relationship with those involved;
- tracking solution patterns around the crisis;
- coming to a consensus on the problem and its goals, including finding a frame to make meaning of it and enlisting action toward its resolution;
- breaking or distancing to gain further perspective for the clients and practitioner;
- initiating the plan and then supporting it; and finally,
- repeatedly summarizing the frame, rationales, goals, and plan; adjusting them as needed; and then reinforcing the shifts as things move forward.

General interventions of the process of change model include the following:

- being flexible to fit frames and rationales to those involved,
- validating the distress and positions of all involved,
- normalizing the distress given the context,
- predicting ongoing patterns,
- positioning the practitioner's orientation to change to empower those involved and to differentiate it from other current vicious cycle patterns,
- offering a frame to make sense of the current crisis and offering a rationale that fits the values and goals of those involved to achieve their goals, and
- prescribing new actions and/or deliberate experiencing of formerly avoided distressing thoughts and situations to initiate support of new pattern shifts.

COMBATING BURNOUT, SECONDARY TRAUMA, AND COMPASSION FATIGUE

Before finishing this work, it is important for us to address the needs of practitioners as they choose to engage with crises as valuable tipping points for transformation in their clients' lives. In service of this, I will turn to a bit of my own history and some positive and cautionary lessons I have drawn from it.

For 14 years, I served as the director of a crisis and brief therapy unit in a large, hospital-based community mental health center (CMHC). Our staff served as essentially the front door of the CMHC: They responded with a therapist on the telephone as clients made their first call for service; scheduled most of the center's first visits with one of our staff within 24 to 48 hours of their request; met with clients as needed for up to 10 sessions; saw people who simply walked in for service; and responded to the hospital's emergency department more than 100 times each month. Some select staff even regularly rode with police and responded to mental health, family, and behavioral emergencies. The center was staffed on-site 24 hours a day, 7 days per week. Most of the cases described in this book were based on experiences of the center's staff members.

Furthermore, the entire crisis/brief therapy staff operated out of the process of change model of intervention championed in this book. As such, all practitioners briefly processed each case with another therapist before meeting each client, took a brief break (when possible) in the midst of each case to process and brainstorm with colleagues, and, finally, debriefed with colleagues upon finishing each case. They were not finished until all of this briefing and debriefing was done. Staff regularly gathered in what we called the "phone room" to back up people answering phones, wait for cases, process cases with colleagues, and engage in mutual support, joke, and often decompress through what might be best termed "dark humor." There was an amazing esprit de corps, joint pride in everyone's expertise, and a remarkable longevity—many staff members stayed together for years. Some referred to the environment of the crisis/brief therapy group as similar to the group on the long-running television series *M*A*S*H*. Fortunately, both the structure of the unit and the process of change model used had built-in components to counteract burnout, secondary traumatization, and compassion fatigue. All of these structures and models of practice were essentially signposts for positive practice that supported both the needs and goals of clients and the needs of all staff involved.

You would think that, as the unit director, I would be sure to always conform to the set structure of processing a case before, during, and after intervention. But one evening, I didn't. I had conducted a very intense first session with a woman and her two teenagers. The family shared how their husband and father had recently "blown his brains out" by shooting himself in front of them. I did good work, but I did not process the case either before, during, or after. Upon arriving home, I sat in my car in the garage and cried my eyes out! This is an example of the danger practitioners face as we choose to seize the opportunity to engage with crises on a more regular basis as I advocate here. The danger for all of us as practitioners is to experience secondary trauma and compassion fatigue, as I did that night.

It may go without saying that many, if not most, of the crises addressed in this book are intense and often traumatic for clients as well as therapists. This frequently leaves practitioners open to what has variously been referred to as burnout, secondary trauma, and compassion fatigue. Again, the full literature is beyond the scope of this final reminder, but we might be best served by turning to much of the work of Charles Figley, who has immersed himself in crisis and trauma, and applied the term *compassion fatigue* to address the potential emotional impact of working with clients in crisis and experiencing trauma (Figley, 2013).

Anyone digging into the emotional impact of working with clients through crisis and trauma will find a rather confusing and overlapping set of terms like *secondary traumatic stress*, *vicarious trauma*, and *burnout*, among others. Each term has slightly different origins and overlapping symptoms, yet all converge on the potential impact on practitioners involved with crises and trauma across a wide array of settings and professions. However, a discussion of the overriding term *compassion fatigue*, its origins and indicators, and the best ways to counteract it may serve us best here. In essence, compassion for the pain and suffering of those we serve is at the heart of crisis intervention. Authentically feeling with our clients is our first step to gaining their trust and building a working alliance to turn the tipping points of their encounters with us toward their goals while supporting their values. We must allow ourselves to be impacted by their lives and often by their trauma. However, as we have mentioned time and again in this book, we as intervenors must resist the draw of being fully pulled into each successive crisis. Failing this, we run the risk of symptoms somewhat similar to those of posttraumatic stress disorder that can spread into our future work through greater detachment from clients, numbness, cynicism, irritability, and growing exhaustion.

Figley referred to compassion fatigue as the "cost of caring" (Figley, 2002). In a classic edited work, he described compassion fatigue as "a state of tension and preoccupation with traumatized patients by re-experiencing the traumatic events, avoidance/numbing of reminders and persistent arousal associated with the patient" (Figley, 2013, p. 1435). More recently, Figley put forward a model that incorporates both risk and resilience factors for compassion fatigue, which helps to summarize the reminders for practitioners and the agencies within which they work (Figley & Figley, 2017; Figley & Ludick, 2017). In this model, exposure to suffering, empathic ability, and empathic concern, along with prolonged exposure to suffering, traumatic memories, and other life demands, contribute to the potential and degree of practitioners developing compassion fatigue. On the other hand and just as importantly, practitioners' self-care, their ability to detach during and outside work, their sense of satisfaction and pride in their work, and the availability of and access to professional and social support within and outside work are all resilience factors. All of these resilience factors were built in at the organizational and individual clinical model levels in the crisis/brief therapy unit described earlier and in the process of change model used by staff there and advocated in this book. All readers are urged to pursue these and other related resources as they move their practice closer to client initial contacts and embrace those tipping points to help *transform* clients' lives as well as preserve the quality of their own. This movement to more rapid intervention and time-effective therapy will confront us all with more crises, as described in this book. Yet if we engage with clients in crisis well, as suggested in the compassion fatigue literature and with the process model of this book, we are likely to develop pride in our compassionate care and in the transformations we see in our clients' lives.

TRACKING THE PROCESS OF CHANGE

Throughout Part II, we have adopted the process of change model to offer a unifying perspective on viewing crises and, consequently, on how best to take advantage of the high motivation for change at these respective tipping points and do crisis intervention in a unifying and effective way. In tracking how the literature has come to describe the characteristic patterns of each different crisis and what have been found to be the most effective approaches to intervention, we have found similar patterns to help unify our understanding of crises and our approach to doing crisis intervention across apparently different crises and different approaches. In terms of unifying effective treatments across approaches, the interested reader is also referred to my previous publication, *Unifying Effective Psychotherapies: Tracing the Process of Change* (Fraser, 2018). That book presents a model (the PROCESS model) that parallels the process of change model advocated here but is applied more broadly to how it unifies *all* effective, evidence-based approaches to therapy across a wide range of problems.

In our present journey, we addressed several crises. We examined trauma as an overriding issue across crises, discussed the paradigm case of suicide as a classic incidental crisis, looked into grief and mourning and its potential interventions as an example of a developmental yet sometimes incidental crisis, and, finally, addressed the endemic examples of crisis in intimate partner violence and sexual assault, showing how their intervention may take two paths (one at the cultural context level, and the other at the individual therapeutic level). A brief overview of each may serve as a helpful reminder.

Trauma as a Common Aspect Across Different Crises

Across all research presented in Chapter 5, the major generic pattern observed around trauma was mastery by avoidance, and most interventions converged on variations of *exposure,* with the exception of present-centered therapy. Although it did not focus on exposure, the present-centered approach interdicted the focus on trauma by acknowledging and validating its distress yet affirming the present and supporting actions to move forward to achieve values and goals. In line with prior work on integrating various effective treatments (Fraser, 2018; Fraser & Solovey, 2007a, 2007b), each of the exposure-based treatments was found to be equally effective, yet each had a different rationale to help make meaning of the trauma and for the paradoxical practice of going toward the painful events that were formerly avoided. All of this is directly in line with the process perspective. Furthermore, by embracing the potential opportunity of the trauma, the research on post-traumatic growth affirmed that trauma has the potential for positive and often transformational outcomes. Recall that the process view suggests that different triggers can lead to the same outcomes, and the same trigger can lead to different outcomes. Remaining open to positive and transformative results can open the door for them to happen.

Suicide as a Potential Incidental Crisis

The major effective interventions for suicidal crises embraced another paradox in the process of change, as described in Chapter 6. Whereas the traditional risk management approach consistently focused on assessing risk and preventing it, all effective interventions started by *affirming* the choice of suicide as a potential way of solving situations that would be described by Chiles and Strosahl (1995) as inescapable, interminable, and intolerable (the three I's). Suicide is not a "thing in itself"; as seen in the social constructivist element of the process view, suicide is a response to a conceived intolerable and painful situation. Although each of several approaches to handling suicide had different premises and rationales, all treated it as an opportunity to try out new and potentially more successful problem-solving options.

Grief and Mourning as a Developmental Crisis

For grief and mourning in Chapter 7, interventions were again turned on their head, as we found that the research suggested that most grieving *did not need intervention*. When practitioners see it as their role to intervene in grief situations that really do not need intervention, they often create more problems than they resolve. Grief, true to the three-sphere process of change working diagram (Figure 4.2), is always shaped by its context, culture, faith-based practices, and traditions. First, the major goal for intervention in grieving is to help only those who are asking for help. Second, grief patterns described as *complex* or *complicated* are the best target for intervention. Once again, rigid adherence to what we have described as first-order solutions in resolving grief (i.e., either rigid denial or rigid immersion in grieving) becomes the focus of intervention. The dual process model of grief resolution, for example, recommends the now familiar position of flexibility, as it *prescribes* that those grieving *deliberately* oscillate between planned times for loss-oriented grieving, times for restoration-oriented activities, and times for rest to avoid overload. These prescriptions for deliberate grieving are a counterintuitive hallmark of most effective grief interventions. Finally, true to the social constructionist aspect of the process model, it is important for all involved with such grief interventions to make space for everyone to make meaning of the loss in their own ways and according to their own traditions.

Intimate Partner Violence as an Endemic Crisis

As an endemic crisis, intimate partner violence is shaped by its cultural context. As we saw in Chapter 8, the influence of power and control are themes cutting across most descriptions of intimate partner violence. The patriarchy and adherence to rigid gender roles have been major focuses of a feminist-based approach to intervention at a cultural level as well as with survivors and perpetrators. However, it must be remembered that, true to the process perspective's concepts of equifinality and multideterminism, not all who adopt rigid gender roles become violent. In addition, intimate violence also occurs in same-sex couples and typically follows similar patterns of power and control, with violence directed toward the partner with less power and control. There are many paths to partner violence. Furthermore, true to the idea that not all solutions that make sense end up solving pressing problems, the interventions of mandatory arrest and feminist-based psycho-educational groups with cognitive behavior therapy overlays have *not* proven effective in the long run. Nevertheless, these approaches continue to be widely applied throughout the United States and other countries (not unlike failing first-order solution patterns repeated over and again). The current research points to focused social advocacy and housing intervention as a priority for survivors before they are able to benefit from group and individual therapy at a cultural level. A relatively recent approach that closely parallels most process-based premises also holds some promise. The Achieving Change Through Values-Based Behavior (ACTV) approach has shown some promising results with batterers and may potentially be equally applied to victims/survivors. The ACTV approach begins by identifying group members' values and goals and then helping each member link those goals with actions that help them build toward those goals in their lives and relationships. The approach assumes that *avoidance* and *attempts to control* uncomfortable thoughts and feelings (termed *experiential avoidance*) only exacerbate those thoughts and feelings and contribute to interpersonal avoidance (a solution-generated vicious cycle). After learning mindfulness to reduce distress and stay in the present, perpetrators are *directed toward* situations typically triggering violence and then helped to reflect on how acting violently does not align with their values and goals (a clear pattern reversal).

On the level of clinical crisis intervention and brief therapy with violence survivors, the main pattern shifts include *validating* distress, *reframing*, and *externalizing* the cause of the attacks to the perpetrators and not the survivor; *positioning* with survivors to encourage their strengths in the face of adversity; clarifying values and goals and *aligning with them*; and then martialing resources and support networks and *empowering* survivors to attend to their safety while moving themselves in *line with their values and goals*. Although such pattern reversals remain challenging in the face of endemic hurdles, progress in shifting these violent cycles has been slow but sure.

Sexual Assault as an Endemic Crisis

As with intimate partner violence, the overall constraints that guide and channel sexual assault are endemic to the cultural sphere—they reside in its norms, language, and positions, as discussed in Chapter 9. Also, as with interpersonal violence (of which sexual assault is a variation), the cultural context has remained resistant and slow to change. In chaos terms, attractors around sexual assault draw perpetrators into positions to take advantage of and have power over their victims. Victims tend to be sexualized as objects for manipulation and assault. Others tend to shame and blame survivors, often disbelieving them or disempowering them by taking control of their safety rather than empowering them as strong survivors in the face of such clear adversity. Cultural constraints create vast underreporting, thus perpetuating the closure of these cycles. Such underreporting is also particularly present for male survivors of sexual assault and for those in same-sex relationships. Interventions at the cultural level converge on opening the systems with new laws and resources. True to process system principles, small shifts often have great ripple effects, like the #MeToo movement. Programmatic reversals in validating, empowering, and supporting survivors include the development of Sexual Assault Nurse Examiner programs in emergency rooms, bystander training to turn the response of others to identifying the assault or its potential as dangerous and interceding, and the support and empowerment resources of the Rape, Abuse & Incest National Network (RAINN). At the clinical level, interventions with survivors all converge on *reframing* the nature of the assault, *externalizing* its source to the perpetrator and not the survivor, *positioning* and thus *empowering* the victim as a strong survivor in the face of adversity, and *reversing* denial and avoidance patterns through *exposure* interventions (again, multiple rationales for interventions converge on the same pattern of often counterintuitive reversals). Finally, in an ongoing affirmation that crises such as sexual assault can also lead to transformative change in positive rather than negative directions, researchers and practitioners have *reversed* their attention from pathologizing the potential outcomes of assaults to instead noticing and supporting *posttraumatic growth*. Marshaling supportive others around the survivor and links with spirituality have been strongly correlated with this new transformative trajectory toward growth.

Convergence

These five crises have been followed as examples of the process of change through their different variations, from incidental, to developmental, to endemic. However, in some ways, the origin of any crisis may vary, as we see in the process of change perspective. What we invariably *do* find is a convergence on repeated failed solutions by all involved around a trigger point, resulting in escalating vicious cycles that form each characteristic crisis. Successful interventions (a) align with the values, goals, culture, and language of those in crisis; (b) identify the vicious cycle patterns; and (c) involve collaboration between the practitioner and those involved to interdict the pattern. Sometimes the efforts are focused at the cultural sphere of our process of change working diagram (Figure 4.2); others are focused on the individuals involved through individual, group, or collateral other interventions; and all involve educating, shifting, and supporting the attitudes and practices of practitioners. If space had allowed in this current work, we might also have addressed other crises such as child sexual abuse, disaster, homicide, and terrorist crises, among others, from the same process-based perspective. Each of these crises and others like them will follow similar common and culturally shaped cycles, with effective interventions recognizing those generic patterns and interdicting, redirecting, and transforming them. Clearly there is more to be said following the thread of the process of change as it links each of these different crisis points. The main point to remember is that those who seek to intervene successfully will need to shift their knowledge and premises on change and the nature of successful intervention to move forward.

CONCLUSIONS AND DIRECTIONS

This work offers a different point of view on the nature of change and the evolution of and intervention in crises. In many ways, this will be a shift for some yet an affirmation for others. What is clear is that embracing this process of change view has a variety of consequences for how we practice, as we discussed in Part I. Approaching crisis intervention from the process of change view involves *adopting the idea of rapid intervention at points of first contact* (whether at a defined crisis point or not) *as a first choice for practice*. Overall, we need to locate ourselves closer to the front door of practice (and even go out that door to meet clients in their own contexts rather than demand they come through *our* doors for help). As we meet clients at these tipping points when they are seeking or needing help, we open windows of opportunity to offer rapid intervention and transformative change unlike what might be there if they were to endure the now common 4- to 6-week waiting lists. Rapid and brief interventions at such crisis points will also likely create greater turnovers in client loads and keep ongoing access for new clients. In line with all of this, we will do well to revisit some of the characteristics of this position, discussed earlier by Budman and Gurman (2002). As we noted in Chapter 3, they viewed doing rapid intervention and time-effective treatment as essentially *a product of a change in point of view*. They suggested that planned rapid intervention and time-limited practitioners tend to (a) value parsimony and least radical interventions, (b) see change as inevitable in a developmental perspective, (c) emphasize client strengths and resources, (d) attempt to initiate change that will continue outside and beyond the end of therapy, (e) maintain focus on the stated problem of the client and agree on resolving it, (f) respect the client's worldview as important to their problem and its resolution, (g) engage with and use resources in clients' lives, and (h) plan and evaluate outcomes (Budman & Gurman, 2002). In line with this, practitioners will need to maintain clear and specific focus, practice higher activity levels, explicitly use time to achieve agreed-upon goals, evaluate progress, engage with outside resources and systems, and keep the door open to future contacts and supports by using an episode-of-care model similar to that of family practitioners (cf. Koss & Shiang, 1994).

ENDINGS AND BEGINNINGS

If this book has managed to achieve its end of opening a window of opportunity for practitioners to view intervention at crisis points as a priority in their practice, it will have achieved some valuable goals. This work aimed to revise the traditional notion of crisis and how to do crisis intervention. Most practitioners across helping disciplines have been taught to assess danger and reduce risks. As an alternative, we have shown how to seize the opportunity of crises as tipping points and to effectively turn them toward rapid resolution and transformative change. Crises are time-limited windows of opportunity to move all involved in new and positive directions in their lives. We have advocated a viewpoint and model for (a) understanding crises in their contexts; (b) engaging with all involved using their values, culture, and language and honoring their goals; and (c) changing vicious cycles into virtuous ones. Finally, following a process of change perspective, we have shown how different types of crises reflect similar vicious cycles and how each of those vicious cycles can be successfully *tipped* toward resolution by embracing the tipping points of crisis as windows of opportunity for rapid intervention and transformative change.

References

Ahrens, C. E., Stansell, J., & Jennings, A. (2010). To tell or not to tell: The impact of disclosure on sexual assault survivors' recovery. *Violence and Victims*, *25*(5), 631–648. https://doi.org/10.1891/0886-6708.25.5.631

Aldwin, C. M. (2009). *Stress, coping, and development: An integrative perspective*. Guilford Press.

Altmaier, E. (2011). Best practices in counseling grief and loss: Finding benefit from trauma. *Journal of Mental Health Counseling*, *33*(1), 33–45. https://doi.org/10.17744/mehc.33.1.tu9wx5w3t2145122

American Psychiatric Association. (2013). *Diagnostic and statistical manual of mental disorders* (5th ed.). https://psycnet.apa.org/doi/10.1176/appi.books.9780890425596

American Psychological Association. (2021, October 19). *Worsening mental health crisis pressures psychologist workforce: 2021 COVID-19 Practitioner Survey*. https://www.apa.org/pubs/reports/practitioner/covid-19-2021

American Psychological Association. (2022). *Post-traumatic stress disorder*. Division 12, Society of Clinical Psychology. https://div12.org/psychological-treatments/disorders/post-traumatic-stress-disorder/

Anderson, B., & Frank, E. (1991). Efficacy of psychological interventions with recent rape victims. In *Rape and sexual assault III: A research handbook* (pp. 75–103). Garland.

APA Presidential Task Force on Evidence-Based Practice. (2006). Evidence-based practice in psychology. *The American Psychologist*, *61*(4), 271–285. https://doi.org/10.1037/0003-066X.61.4.271

Barlow, D. H. (Ed.). (2021). *Clinical handbook of psychological disorders: A step-by-step treatment manual*. Guilford Press.

Barner, J. R., & Carney, M. M. (2011). Interventions for intimate partner violence: A historical review. *Journal of Family Violence*, *26*(3), 235–244. https://doi.org/10.1007/s10896-011-9359-3

Basile, K. C., Smith, S. G., Kresnow, M., Khatiwada, S., & Leemis, R. W. (2022). *The National Intimate Partner and Sexual Violence Survey: 2016/2017 report on sexual violence*. Centers for Disease Control and Prevention.

Bateson, G. (1978). Steps to an ecology of mind. In *Collected essays in anthropology, psychiatry, evolution, an epistemology*. Ballantine Books.

Bateson, G. (1979). *Mind and nature: A necessary unity*. Dutton.

Beck, J. S. (2005). *Cognitive therapy for challenging problems: What to do when the basics don't work*. Guilford Press.

Benish, S. G., Imel, Z. E., & Wampold, B. E. (2008). The relative efficacy of bona fide psychotherapies for treating post-traumatic stress disorder: A meta-analysis of direct comparisons. *Clinical Psychology Review, 28*(5), 746–758. https://doi.org/10.1016/j.cpr.2007.10.005

Berta, M., & Zarling, A. (2019). A preliminary examination of an acceptance and commitment therapy-based program for incarcerated domestic violence offenders. *Violence and Victims, 34*(2), 213–228. https://doi.org/10.1891/0886-6708.VV-D-17-00106

Berwick, D. M. (2002). *Escape fire: Lessons for the future of health care*. Commonwealth Fund.

Bonanno, G. A., & Lilienfeld, S. O. (2008). Let's be realistic: When grief counseling is effective and when it's not. *Professional Psychology: Research and Practice, 39*(3), 377–378. https://doi.org/10.1037/0735-7028.39.3.377

Bowlby, J. (1969). *Attachment and loss*. Random House.

Bowlby, J. (2005). *A secure base: Clinical applications of attachment theory* (Vol. 393). Taylor & Francis.

Bradley, R., Greene, J., Russ, E., Dutra, L., & Westen, D. (2005). A multidimensional meta-analysis of psychotherapy for PTSD. *The American Journal of Psychiatry, 162*(2), 214–227. https://doi.org/10.1176/appi.ajp.162.2.214

Brewin, C. R., Dalgleish, T., & Joseph, S. (1996). A dual representation theory of posttraumatic stress disorder. *Psychological Review, 103*(4), 670–686. https://doi.org/10.1037/0033-295x.103.4.670

Briggs, J., & Peat, F. D. (1989). *Turbulent mirror: An illustrated guide to chaos theory and the science of wholeness*. Harper Collins Publishers.

Briggs, J., & Peat, F. D. (2000). *Seven life lessons of chaos: Spiritual wisdom from the science of change*. Harper Perennial.

Bryan, C. J. (2021). *Rethinking suicide: Why prevention fails, and how we can do better*. Oxford University Press. https://doi.org/10.1093/med-psych/9780190050634.001.0001

Buckley, W. (1967). *Sociology and modern systems theory*. Prentice-Hall.

Budman, S. H., & Gurman, A. S. (2002). *Theory and practice of brief therapy*. Guilford Press.

Burgess, A. W., & Holmstrom, L. L. (1974). Rape trauma syndrome. *The American Journal of Psychiatry, 131*(9), 981–986. https://doi.org/10.1176/ajp.131.9.981

Caldwell, J. E., Swan, S. C., & Woodbrown, V. D. (2012). Gender differences in intimate partner violence outcomes. *Psychology of Violence, 2*(1), 42–57. https://doi.org/10.1037/a0026296

Calhoun, L. G., & Tedeschi, R. G. (2014a). The foundations of posttraumatic growth: An expanded framework. In L. G. Calhoun & R. G. Tedeschi (Eds.), *Handbook of posttraumatic growth* (pp. 3–23). Routledge.

Calhoun, L. G., & Tedeschi, R. G. (2014b). *Handbook of posttraumatic growth: Research and practice*. Routledge. https://doi.org/10.4324/9781315805597

Campbell, R. (2005). What really happened? A validation study of rape survivors' help-seeking experiences with the legal and medical systems. *Violence and Victims, 20*(1), 55–68. https://doi.org/10.1891/vivi.2005.20.1.55

Campbell, R., Bybee, D., Townsend, S. M., Shaw, J., Karim, N., & Markowitz, J. (2014). The impact of Sexual Assault Nurse Examiner programs on criminal justice case outcomes: A multisite replication study. *Violence Against Women, 20*(5), 607–625. https://doi.org/10.1177/1077801214536286

Campbell, R., Patterson, D., & Lichty, L. F. (2005). The effectiveness of Sexual Assault Nurse Examiner (SANE) programs: A review of psychological, medical, legal, and community outcomes. *Trauma, Violence, & Abuse, 6*(4), 313–329. https://doi.org/10.1177/1524838005280328

Cann, A., Calhoun, L. G., Tedeschi, R. G., & Solomon, D. T. (2010). Posttraumatic growth and depreciation as independent experiences and predictors of well-being. *Journal of Loss and Trauma, 15*(3), 151–166. https://doi.org/10.1080/15325020903375826

Caplan, G. (1963). Emotional crises. In T. Alexander (Ed.), *The encyclopedia of mental health* (Vol. II, pp. 521–532). Franklin Watts. https://doi.org/10.1037/11549-015

Caplan, G., & Caplan, R. (2000). Principles of community psychiatry. *Community Mental Health Journal, 36*(1), 7–24. https://doi.org/10.1023/A:1001894709715

Caplan, G. E. (1961). *Prevention of mental disorders in children: Initial explorations*. Basic Books. https://doi.org/10.1097/00000441-196111000-00043

Capra, F. (Director). (1946). *It's a wonderful life* [Film]. Paramount.

Carr, D. (2023, July 31). Trauma: America's favorite diagnosis. *New York Magazine*.

Carver, C. S., & Scheier, M. F. (1982). Control theory: A useful conceptual framework for personality-social, clinical, and health psychology. *Psychological Bulletin, 92*(1), 111–135. https://doi.org/10.1037/0033-2909.92.1.111

Carver, C. S., & Scheier, M. F. (2000). Autonomy and self-regulation. *Psychological Inquiry, 11*(4), 284–291.

Cavaiola, A. A., & Colford, J. E. (2017). *Crisis intervention: A practical guide*. Sage.

Chattopadhyay, P., Glick, W. H., & Huber, G. P. (2001). Organizational actions in response to threats and opportunities. *Academy of Management Journal, 44*(5), 937–955. https://doi.org/10.2307/3069439

Chiles, J. A., & Strosahl, K. D. (1995). *The suicidal patient: Principles of assessment, treatment, and case management*. American Psychiatric Association.

Cholbi, M. (2010). A Kantian defense of prudential suicide. *Journal of Moral Philosophy, 7*(4), 489–515.

Clay, R. A. (2023, January 1). Suicide prevention gets a new lifeline. *Monitor on Psychology, 54*(1), 73. https://www.apa.org/monitor/2023/01/trends-suicide-prevention-lifeline

Condino, V., Tanzilli, A., Speranza, A. M., & Lingiardi, V. (2016). Therapeutic interventions in intimate partner violence: An overview. *Research in Psychotherapy, 19*(2), 79–88. https://doi.org/10.4081/ripppo.2016.241

Constantino, M. J., & Bernecker, S. L. (2014). Bridging the common factors and empirically supported treatment camps: Comment on Laska, Gurman, and Wampold. *Psychotherapy, 51*(4), 505–509. https://doi.org/10.1037/a0036604

Covers, M. L. V., de Jongh, A., Huntjens, R. J. C., de Roos, C., van den Hout, M., & Bicanic, I. A. E. (2021). Early intervention with eye movement desensitization and reprocessing (EMDR) therapy to reduce the severity of post-traumatic stress symptoms in recent rape victims: A randomized controlled trial. *European Journal of Psychotraumatology, 12*(1), 1943188. https://doi.org/10.1080/20008198.2021.1943188

Currier, J. M., Holland, J. M., & Neimeyer, R. A. (2006). Sense-making, grief, and the experience of violent loss: Toward a mediational model. *Death Studies, 30*(5), 403–428. https://doi.org/10.1080/07481180600614351

Currier, J. M., Neimeyer, R. A., & Berman, J. S. (2008). The effectiveness of psychotherapeutic interventions for bereaved persons: A comprehensive quantitative review. *Psychological Bulletin, 134*(5), 648–661. https://doi.org/10.1037/0033-2909.134.5.648

Davis, C. G., Nolen-Hoeksema, S., & Larson, J. (1998). Making sense of loss and benefiting from the experience: Two construals of meaning. *Journal of Personality and Social Psychology, 75*(2), 561–574. https://doi.org/10.1037/0022-3514.75.2.561

de Shazer, S. (1991). *Putting difference to work.* W. W. Norton.

Dhungel, B., Shand, F., Nguyen, P., Wang, Y., Fujita-Imazu, S., Khin Maung Soe, J., Xie, J., Wang, X., Li, J., & Gilmour, S. (2023). Method-specific suicide mortality in the United States in the 21st century. *Annals of Internal Medicine, 177*(1), 110–113. https://doi.org/10.7326/M23-2533

Doka, K. J., & Martin, T. L. (2011). *Grieving beyond gender: Understanding the ways men and women mourn.* Routledge. https://doi.org/10.4324/9780203886069

Duncan, B. L., Miller, S. D., Wampold, B. E., & Hubble, M. A. (Eds.). (2010). *The heart and soul of change: Delivering what works in therapy* (2nd ed.). American Psychological Association. https://doi.org/10.1037/12075-000

Durkheim, E. (2005). *Suicide: A study in sociology.* Routledge. https://doi.org/10.4324/9780203994320

Dworkin, E. R., & Schumacher, J. A. (2018). Preventing posttraumatic stress related to sexual assault through early intervention: A systematic review. *Trauma, Violence, & Abuse, 19*(4), 459–472. https://doi.org/10.1177/1524838016669518

Eckhardt, C. I., Murphy, C. M., Whitaker, D. J., Sprunger, J., Dykstra, R., & Woodard, K. (2013). The effectiveness of intervention programs for perpetrators and victims of intimate partner violence. *Partner Abuse, 4*(2), 196–231. https://doi.org/10.1891/1946-6560.4.2.196

Ehlers, A., & Clark, D. M. (2000). A cognitive model of posttraumatic stress disorder. *Behaviour Research and Therapy, 38*(4), 319–345. https://doi.org/10.1016/s0005-7967(99)00123-0

Encyclopedia Britannica. (n.d.). *Catastrophe theory.* Retrieved February 20, 2023, from https://www.britannica.com/science/catastrophe-theory-mathematics

Ericksen, J., Dudley, C., McIntosh, G., Ritch, L., Shumay, S., & Simpson, M. (2002). Clients' experiences with a specialized sexual assault service. *Journal of Emergency Nursing, 28*(1), 86–90. https://doi.org/10.1067/men.2002.121740

Farberow, N. L., & Shneidman, E. S. (1961). *The cry for help.* McGraw-Hill.

Fennell, M. J., & Teasdale, J. D. (1987). Cognitive therapy for depression: Individual differences and the process of change. *Cognitive Therapy and Research, 11*(2), 253–271. https://doi.org/10.1007/BF01183269

Figley, C. R. (1988). A five-phase treatment of post-traumatic stress disorder in families. *Journal of Traumatic Stress, 1,* 127–141.

Figley, C. R. (2002). Compassion fatigue: Psychotherapists' chronic lack of self care. *Journal of Clinical Psychology, 58*(11), 1433–1441. https://doi.org/10.1002/jclp.10090

Figley, C. R. (2013). *Compassion fatigue: Coping with secondary traumatic stress disorder in those who treat the traumatized.* Routledge.

Figley, C. R., & Figley, K. R. (2017). Compassion fatigue resilience. *The Oxford handbook of compassion science* (pp. 387–398). Oxford University Press.

Figley, C. R., & Ludick, M. (2017). Secondary traumatization and compassion fatigue. In S. N. Gold (Ed.), *APA handbook of trauma psychology: Foundations in knowledge* (pp. 573–593). American Psychological Association. https://doi.org/10.1037/0000019-029

Fiore, J. (2021). A systematic review of the dual process model of coping with bereavement (1999–2016). *Omega: Journal of Death and Dying, 84*(2), 414–458. https://doi.org/10.1177/0030222819893139

Fischer, P., Krueger, J. I., Greitemeyer, T., Vogrincic, C., Kastenmüller, A., Frey, D., Heene, M., Wicher, M., & Kainbacher, M. (2011). The bystander-effect: A meta-analytic review on bystander intervention in dangerous and non-dangerous emergencies. *Psychological Bulletin, 137*(4), 517–537. https://doi.org/10.1037/a0023304

Foa, E. B., McLean, C. P., Zang, Y., Rosenfield, D., Yadin, E., Yarvis, J. S., Mintz, J., Young-McCaughan, S., Borah, E. V., Dondanville, K. A., Fina, B. A., Hall-Clark, B. N., Lichner, T., Litz, B. T., Roache, J., Wright, E. C., Peterson, A. L., & Strong Star Consortium. (2018). Effect of prolonged exposure therapy delivered over 2 weeks vs 8 weeks vs present-centered therapy on PTSD symptom severity in military personnel: A randomized clinical trial. *JAMA, 319*(4), 354–364. https://doi.org/10.1001/jama.2017.21242

Frank, J. D., & Frank, J. B. (1991). *Persuasion and healing: A comparative study of psychotherapy* (3rd ed.). Johns Hopkins University Press.

Fraser, J. S. (1986). The crisis interview: Strategic rapid intervention. *Journal of Strategic and Systemic Therapies, 5*(3 & 4), 71–87.

Fraser, J. S. (1988). Strategic rapid intervention in wife beating. In E. W. Nunnally, C. S. Chilman, & F. M. Cox (Eds.), *Troubled relationships* (pp. 163–191). Sage.

Fraser, J. S. (1989). The strategic rapid intervention approach. In C. Figley (Ed.), *Treating stress in families* (pp. 122–157). Brunner/Mazel.

Fraser, J. S. (1995a). Process, problems, and solutions in brief therapy. *Journal of Marital and Family Therapy, 21*(3), 265–279. https://doi.org/10.1111/j.1752-0606.1995.tb00161.x

Fraser, J. S. (1995b). Solution focused therapy—As a problem. In W. Ray & S. de Shazer (Eds.), *Evolving brief therapies: Essays in honor of John Weakland*. Geist & Russell.

Fraser, J. S. (1995c). Strategic rapid intervention: Constructing the process of rapid change. In J. Weakland & W. Ray (Eds.), *Propagations: Thirty years of influence of the Mental Research Institute* (pp. 211–235). Haworth Press.

Fraser, J. S. (1998a). A catalyst model: Guidelines for doing crisis intervention and brief therapy from a process view. *Crisis Intervention and Time-Limited Treatment, 4*(2–3), 159–177.

Fraser, J. S. (1998b). A process view of crisis and crisis intervention: Critique and reformulation. *Crisis Intervention and Time-Limited Treatment, 4*(2–3), 125–143.

Fraser, J. S. (2001). Crisis, chaos, and brief therapy: Constructive interventions in high-risk situations. In L. VandeCreek & T. L. Jackson (Eds.), *Innovations in clinical practice: A source book* (Vol. 19, pp. 95–111). Professional Resource Press.

Fraser, J. S. (2018). *Unifying effective psychotherapies: Tracing the process of change*. American Psychological Association. https://doi.org/10.1037/0000078-000

Fraser, J. S. (2020). The crisis interview: Strategic rapid intervention. *Journal of Systemic Therapies, 39*(2), 65–83. https://doi.org/10.1521/jsyt.2020.39.2.65

Fraser, J. S., & Solovey, A. (2007a). *Brief therapy: The process of change and episodes of care*. Scientist-Practitioner.com. https://corescholar.libraries.wright.edu/sopp/118/

Fraser, J. S., & Solovey, A. D. (2007b). *Second-order change in psychotherapy: The golden thread that unifies effective treatments*. American Psychological Association. https://doi.org/10.1037/11499-000

Freud, S. (1917). Mourning and melancholia. In *Essential papers on depression*. New York University Press.

Freud, S. (1922). Mourning and melancholia. *Journal of Nervous and Mental Disease, 56*(5), 543–545. https://doi.org/10.1097/00005053-192211000-00066

Friedman, R., & James, J. W. (2009, March). The myth of the stages of grieving, death, and grief. *Counseling Today*, 48–52.

Frost, N. D., Laska, K. M., & Wampold, B. E. (2014). The evidence for present-centered therapy as a treatment for posttraumatic stress disorder. *Journal of Traumatic Stress, 27*(1), 1–8. https://doi.org/10.1002/jts.21881

Gergen, K. J. (1985). The social constructionist movement in modern psychology. *American Psychologist, 40*(3), 266–275. https://doi.org/10.1037/0003-066X.40.3.266

Gergen, K. J. (2022). *An invitation to social construction: Co-creating the future.* Sage.

Gersen, J. S. (2023, March 29). Revisiting the Brock Turner case. *The New Yorker.* https://www.newyorker.com/news/our-columnists/revisiting-the-brock-turner-case

Gladwell, M. (2006). *The tipping point: How little things can make a big difference.* Little, Brown and Company.

Glass, N. E., Clough, A., Messing, J. T., Bloom, T., Brown, M. L., Eden, K. B., Campbell, J. C., Gielen, A., Laughon, K., Grace, K. T., Turner, R. M., Alvarez, C., Case, J., Barnes-Hoyt, J., Alhusen, J., Hanson, G. C., & Perrin, N. A. (2022). Longitudinal impact of the myPlan App on health and safety among college women experiencing partner violence. *Journal of Interpersonal Violence, 37*(13–14), NP11436–NP11459. https://doi.org/10.1177/0886260521991880

Gleick, J. (2008). *Chaos: Making a new science.* Penguin.

Goerner, S. (1995). Chaos, evolution, and deep ecology. In R. Robertson & A. Combs (Eds.), *Chaos theory in psychology and the life sciences* (pp. 17–38). Psychology Press. https://doi.org/10.4324/9781315806280-3

Gondolf, E. W. (2002). *Batterer intervention systems: Issues, outcomes, and recommendations.* Sage.

Gondolf, E. W. (2012). *The future of batterer programs: Reassessing evidence-based practice.* Northeastern University Press.

Goolishian, H. A., & Winderman, L. (1988). Constructivism, autopoiesis and problem determined systems. *The Irish Journal of Psychology, 9*(1), 130–143. https://doi.org/10.1080/03033910.1988.10557710

Gornick, J., Burt, M. R., & Pittman, K. J. (1985). Structure and activities of rape crisis centers in the early 1980s. *Crime and Delinquency, 31*(2), 247–268. https://doi.org/10.1177/0011128785031002006

Gould, S. J., & Eldredge, N. (1972). Punctuated equilibria: An alternative to phyletic gradualism. *Models in paleobiology* (pp. 82–115). Freeman, Cooper & Company.

Graham, D. L., Rawlings, E. I., Ihms, K., Latimer, D., Foliano, J., Thompson, A., Suttman, K., Farrington, M., & Hacker, R. (1995). A scale for identifying "Stockholm syndrome" reactions in young dating women: Factor structure, reliability, and validity. *Violence and Victims, 10*(1), 3–22. https://doi.org/10.1891/0886-6708.10.1.3

Grant, A. (2021). *Think again: The power of knowing what you don't know.* Penguin.

Groleau, J. M., Calhoun, L. G., Cann, A., & Tedeschi, R. G. (2013). The role of centrality of events in posttraumatic distress and posttraumatic growth. *Psychological Trauma: Theory, Research, Practice, and Policy, 5*(5), 477–483. https://doi.org/10.1037/a0028809

Hackett, S., McWhirter, P. T., & Lesher, S. (2016). The therapeutic efficacy of domestic violence: Victim interventions. *Trauma, Violence & Abuse, 17*(2), 123–132. https://doi.org/10.1177/1524838014566720

Hayes, S. C., Pistorello, J., & Levin, M. E. (2012). Acceptance and commitment therapy as a unified model of behavior change. *The Counseling Psychologist, 40*(7), 976–1002. https://doi.org/10.1002/wps.20626

Hembree, E. A., Foa, E. B., Dorfan, N. M., Street, G. P., Kowalski, J., & Tu, X. (2003). Do patients drop out prematurely from exposure therapy for PTSD? *Journal of Traumatic Stress, 16*(6), 555–562. https://doi.org/10.1023/B:JOTS. 0000004078.93012.7d

Hinton, D. (2015). *Tao te ching*. Catapult.

Hoppe, S. J., Zhang, Y., Hayes, B. E., & Bills, M. A. (2020). Mandatory arrest for domestic violence and repeat offending: A meta-analysis. *Aggression and Violent Behavior, 53*, 101430. https://doi.org/10.1016/j.avb.2020.101430

Horvath, A. O., Del Re, A. C., Flückiger, C., & Symonds, D. (2011). Alliance in individual psychotherapy. *Psychotherapy, 48*(1), 9–16. https://doi.org/ 10.1037/a0022186

Howard, K. I., Kopta, S. M., Krause, M. S., & Orlinsky, D. E. (1986). The dose-effect relationship in psychotherapy. *American Psychologist, 41*(2), 159–164. https://doi.org/10.1037/0003-066X.41.2.159

Howard, K. I., Lueger, R. J., Maling, M. S., & Martinovich, Z. (1993). A phase model of psychotherapy outcome: Causal mediation of change. *Journal of Consulting and Clinical Psychology, 61*(4), 678–685. https://doi.org/10.1037/ 0022-006X.61.4.678

Humphrey, K. M. (2009). *Counseling strategies for loss and grief*. American Counseling Association.

Imel, Z. E., Laska, K., Jakupcak, M., & Simpson, T. L. (2013). Meta-analysis of dropout in treatments for posttraumatic stress disorder. *Journal of Consulting and Clinical Psychology, 81*(3), 394–404. https://doi.org/10.1037/ a0031474

Interlandi, J. (2014, May 22). A revolutionary approach to treating PTSD. *The New York Times*. https://www.nytimes.com/2014/05/25/magazine/ a-revolutionary-approach-to-treating-ptsd.html

International Women's Day. (2024). *About International Women's Day*. https:// www.internationalwomensday.com/About

James, R. K., & Gilliland, B. E. (2016). *Crisis intervention strategies*. Cengage Learning.

Janoff-Bulman, R. (2004). Posttraumatic growth: Three explanatory models. *Psychological Inquiry, 15*(1), 30–34.

Janoff-Bulman, R. (2010). *Shattered assumptions*. Simon and Schuster.

Jobes, D. A. (2016). *Managing suicidal risk: A collaborative approach*. Guilford Press.

Johnson, D. M., & Zlotnick, C. (2009). HOPE for battered women with PTSD in domestic violence shelters. *Professional Psychology: Research and Practice, 40*(3), 234–241. https://doi.org/10.1037/a0012519

Joiner, T. E., Jr., Van Orden, K. A., Witte, T. K., & Rudd, M. D. (2009). *The interpersonal theory of suicide: Guidance for working with suicidal clients*. American Psychological Association. https://doi.org/10.1037/11869-000

Joseph, S., Linley, P. A., & Harris, G. J. (2004). Understanding positive change following trauma and adversity: Structural clarification. *Journal of Loss and Trauma, 10*(1), 83–96. https://doi.org/10.1080/15325020490890741

Kahneman, D. (2011). *Thinking, fast and slow*. Farrar, Straus & Giroux.

Kahneman, D., & Tversky, A. (2013). Prospect theory: An analysis of decision under risk. In *Handbook of the fundamentals of financial decision making: Part I* (pp. 99–127). World Scientific. https://doi.org/10.1142/9789814417358_0006

Kanel, K. (2019). *A guide to crisis intervention* (6th ed.). Cengage Learning.

Kastenbaum, R., & Thuell, S. (1995). Cookies baking, coffee brewing: Toward a contextual theory of dying. *Omega: Journal of Death and Dying, 31*(3), 175–187. https://doi.org/10.2190/LQPX-71DE-V5AA-EPFT

Kennedy, A. C., & Prock, K. A. (2018). "I still feel like I am not normal": A review of the role of stigma and stigmatization among female survivors of child sexual abuse, sexual assault, and intimate partner violence. *Trauma, Violence, & Abuse, 19*(5), 512–527. https://doi.org/10.1177/1524838016673601

Kennedy, J. F. (1959, April 12). *Convocation of the United Negro College Fund* [Speech].

Kessler, R. C., Chiu, W. T., Demler, O., & Walters, E. E. (2005). Prevalence, severity, and comorbidity of 12-month *DSM-IV* disorders in the National Comorbidity Survey Replication. *Archives of General Psychiatry, 62*(6), 617–627. https://doi.org/10.1001/archpsyc.62.6.617

Kimble, C., & Chettiar, I. M. (2018, October 4). *Sexual assault remains dramatically underreported*. Brennan Center for Justice. https://www.brennancenter.org/our-work/analysis-opinion/sexual-assault-remains-dramatically-underreported?GA_loc_physical_ms=9026941

Kitchens, C. (2014, March 20). It's time to end 'rape culture' hysteria. *Time*. https://time.com/30545/its-time-to-end-rape-culture-hysteria/

Konigsberg, R. D. (2011). *The truth about grief: The myth of its five stages and the new science of loss*. Simon and Schuster.

Koss, M. P., Abbey, A., Campbell, R., Cook, S., Norris, J., Testa, M., Ullman, S., West, C., & White, J. (2007). Revising the SES: A collaborative process to improve assessment of sexual aggression and victimization. *Psychology of Women Quarterly, 31*(4), 357–370. https://doi.org/10.1111/j.1471-6402.2007.00385.x

Koss, M. P., & Shiang, J. (1994). Research on brief psychotherapy. In A. E. Bergin & S. L. Garfield (Eds.), *Handbook of psychotherapy and behavior change* (pp. 664–700). John Wiley & Sons.

Koss, M. P., White, J. W., & Lopez, E. C. (2017). Victim voice in reenvisioning responses to sexual and physical violence nationally and internationally. *American Psychologist, 72*(9), 1019–1030. https://doi.org/10.1037/amp0000233

Kubany, E. S., Hill, E. E., & Owens, J. A. (2003). Cognitive trauma therapy for battered women with PTSD: Preliminary findings. *Journal of Traumatic Stress, 16*, 81–91. https://doi.org/10.1023/A:1022019629803

Kubany, E. S., Hill, E. E., Owens, J. A., Iannce-Spencer, C., McCaig, M. A., Tremayne, K. J., & Williams, P. L. (2004). Cognitive trauma therapy for battered women with PTSD (CTT-BW). *Journal of Consulting and Clinical Psychology, 72*(1), 3–18. https://doi.org/10.1037/0022-006X.72.1.3

Kübler-Ross, E. (1969). *On death and dying*. Macmillan.

Lakoff, G. (2014). *The all new don't think of an elephant! Know your values and frame the debate*. Chelsea Green Publishing.

Lang, P. J. (1977). Imagery in therapy: An information processing analysis of fear. *Behavior Therapy, 8*, 862–886. https://doi.org/10.1016/j.beth.2016.08.011

Laska, K. M., Gurman, A. S., & Wampold, B. E. (2014). Expanding the lens of evidence-based practice in psychotherapy: A common factors perspective. *Psychotherapy, 51*(4), 467–481. https://doi.org/10.1037/a0034332

Lawrence, E., Mazurek, C., & Reardon, K. W. (2021). Comparing recidivism rates among domestically violent men enrolled in ACTV versus Duluth/CBT. *Journal of Consulting and Clinical Psychology, 89*(5), 469–475. https://doi.org/10.1037/ccp0000649

Lester, D. (2013). Right-to-die organizations. In D. Lester (Ed.), *Suicide prevention: Resources for the millennium* (pp. 285–298). Routledge.

Levy, R., & Mattsson, M. (2023, April 27). *The effects of social movements: Evidence from #MeToo*. SSRN. https://ssrn.com/abstract=3496903

Lindemann, E. (1944). Symptomatology and management of acute grief. *The American Journal of Psychiatry, 101*(2), 141–148. https://doi.org/10.1176/ajp.101.2.141

Linehan, M. (2014). *DBT skills training manual*. Guilford Press.

Linehan, M. M., Korslund, K. E., Harned, M. S., Gallop, R. J., Lungu, A., Neacsiu, A. D., McDavid, J., Comtois, K. A., & Murray-Gregory, A. M. (2015). Dialectical behavior therapy for high suicide risk in individuals with borderline personality disorder: A randomized clinical trial and component analysis. *JAMA Psychiatry, 72*(5), 475–482. https://doi.org/10.1001/jamapsychiatry.2014.3039

Linley, P. A., & Joseph, S. (2004a). Applied positive psychology: A new perspective for professional practice. In P. A. Linley & S. Joseph (Eds.), *Positive psychology in practice* (pp. 3–12). John Wiley & Sons.

Linley, P. A., & Joseph, S. (2004b). Positive change following trauma and adversity: A review. *Journal of Traumatic Stress, 17*(1), 11–21. https://doi.org/10.1023/B:JOTS.0000014671.27856.7e

Linley, P. A., & Joseph, S. (2005). The human capacity for growth through adversity. *American Psychologist, 60*(3), 262–264. https://doi.org/10.1037/0003-066X.60.3.262b

Linley, P. A., Joseph, S., Harrington, S., & Wood, A. M. (2006). Positive psychology: Past, present, and (possible) future. *The Journal of Positive Psychology, 1*(1), 3–16. https://doi.org/10.1080/17439760500372796

Lomax, J., & Meyrick, J. (2022). Effectiveness of psychosocial interventions on wellbeing outcomes for adolescent or adult victim/survivors of recent rape or sexual assault. *Journal of Health Psychology, 27*(2), 305–331. https://doi.org/10.1177/1359105320950799

Lorenz, K. (2021). *On aggression.* Routledge.

Maercker, A., & Zoellner, T. (2004). The Janus face of self-perceived growth: Toward a two-component model of posttraumatic growth. *Psychological Inquiry, 15*(1), 41–48.

Maier, S. F., & Seligman, M. E. (1976). Learned helplessness: Theory and evidence. *Journal of Experimental Psychology: General, 105*(1), 3–46. https://doi.org/10.1037/0096-3445.105.1.3

Mair, V. H. (2009). *How a misunderstanding about Chinese characters has led many astray.* Pinyin. https://pinyin.info/chinese/crisis.html

Martin, P. Y. (2013). *Rape work: Victims, gender, and emotions in organization and community context.* Routledge. https://doi.org/10.4324/9780203614457

Martin, T. L., & Doka, K. J. (2000). *Men don't cry—Women do: Transcending gender stereotypes of grief.* Brunner-Mazel.

Maxwell, Z. (2014, March 27). Rape culture is real. *Time.* https://time.com/40110/rape-culture-is-real/

McCloskey, K. A., & Fraser, J. S. (1997). Using feminist MRI brief therapy during initial contact with victims of domestic violence. *Psychotherapy: Theory, Research, Practice, Training, 34*(4), 433–446. https://doi.org/10.1037/h0087653

McDonagh, A., Friedman, M., McHugo, G., Ford, J., Sengupta, A., Mueser, K., Demment, C. C., Fournier, D., Schnurr, P. P., & Descamps, M. (2005). Randomized trial of cognitive-behavioral therapy for chronic posttraumatic stress disorder in adult female survivors of childhood sexual abuse. *Journal of Consulting and Clinical Psychology, 73*(3), 515–524. https://doi.org/10.1037/0022-006X.73.3.515

McLean, C. P., & Foa, E. B. (2011). Prolonged exposure therapy for post-traumatic stress disorder: A review of evidence and dissemination. *Expert Review of Neurotherapeutics, 11*(8), 1151–1163. https://doi.org/10.1586/ern.11.94

McLeod, D. A., Havig, K., Natale, A., & Pharris, A. (2020). Intimate partner violence: Innovations in theory to inform clinical practice, policy, and research. *Social Sciences, 9*(5), 71. https://doi.org/10.3390/socsci9050071

McMahon, S. M. (2019). History of the anti-rape movement. In W. T. O'Donohue & P. A. Schewe (Eds.), *Handbook of sexual assault and sexual assault prevention* (pp. 47–53). Springer, Cham. https://doi.org/10.1007/978-3-030-23645-8_3

Merriam-Webster. (n.d.-a). Fractal. In *Merriam-Webster.com dictionary.* Retrieved October 1, 2024, from https://www.merriam-webster.com/dictionary/fractal#-dictionary-entry-1

Merriam-Webster. (n.d.-b). Patriarchy. In *Merriam-Webster.com dictionary*. Retrieved October 27, 2023, from https://www.merriam-webster.com/dictionary/patriarchy

Messing, J. T., Ward-Lasher, A., Thaller, J., & Bagwell-Gray, M. E. (2015). The state of intimate partner violence intervention: Progress and continuing challenges. *Social Work*, *60*(4), 305–313. https://doi.org/10.1093/sw/swv027

Michael, T., Halligan, S. L., Clark, D. M., & Ehlers, A. (2007). Rumination in post-traumatic stress disorder. *Depression and Anxiety*, *24*(5), 307–317. https://doi.org/10.1002/da.20228

Michel, K. E., & Jobes, D. A. (2011). *Building a therapeutic alliance with the suicidal patient*. American Psychological Association. https://doi.org/10.1037/12303-000

Micklitz, H. M., Glass, C. M., Bengel, J., & Sander, L. B. (2024). Efficacy of psychosocial interventions for survivors of intimate partner violence: A systematic review and meta-analysis. *Trauma, Violence & Abuse*, *25*(2), 1000–1017. https://doi.org/10.1177/15248380231169481

Miles, L. W., Valentine, J. L., Mabey, L. J., Hopkins, E. S., Stodtmeister, P. J., Rockwood, R. B., & Moxley, A. N. H. (2024). A systematic review of evidence-based treatments for adolescent and adult sexual assault victims. *Journal of the American Psychiatric Nurses Association*, *30*(3), 480–502. https://doi.org/10.1177/10783903231216138

Miller, C. (2020). *Know my name: A memoir*. Penguin.

Miller, M. C. (1999). Suicide-prevention contracts: Advantages, disadvantages, and an alternative approach. In D. G. Jacobs (Ed.), *The Harvard Medical School guide to suicide assessment and intervention* (pp. 463–481). Jossey-Bass/Wiley.

Mowrer, O. H. (1960). Two-factor learning theory: Versions one and two. In O. H. Mowrer (Ed.), *Learning theory and behavior* (pp. 63–91). John Wiley & Sons Inc. https://doi.org/10.1037/10802-003

Mujal, G. N., Taylor, M. E., Fry, J. L., Gochez-Kerr, T. H., & Weaver, N. L. (2021). A systematic review of bystander interventions for the prevention of sexual violence. *Trauma, Violence, & Abuse*, *22*(2), 381–396. https://doi.org/10.1177/1524838019849587

Murphy-Oikonen, J., McQueen, K., Miller, A., Chambers, L., & Hiebert, A. (2022). Unfounded sexual assault: Women's experiences of not being believed by the police. *Journal of Interpersonal Violence*, *37*(11–12), NP8916–NP8940. https://doi.org/10.1177/0886260520978190

National Council of Mental Wellbeing. (2022, February 18). *2021 CCBHC State Impact Report: Transforming state behavioral health systems*. https://www.thenationalcouncil.org/resources/2021-ccbhc-state-impact-report-transforming-state-behavioral-health-systems/

Neimeyer, R. A. (2000). Searching for the meaning of meaning: Grief therapy and the process of reconstruction. *Death Studies*, *24*(6), 541–558. https://doi.org/10.1080/07481180050121480

Neimeyer, R. A. (2001). *Meaning reconstruction & the experience of loss*. American Psychological Association. https://doi.org/10.1037/10397-000

Neimeyer, R. A., & Currier, J. M. (2009). Grief therapy: Evidence of efficacy and emerging directions. *Current Directions in Psychological Science, 18*(6), 352–356. https://doi.org/10.1111/j.1467-8721.2009.01666.x

Neimeyer, R. A., Klass, D., & Dennis, M. R. (2014). A social constructionist account of grief: Loss and the narration of meaning. *Death Studies, 38*(8), 485–498. https://doi.org/10.1080/07481187.2014.913454

Nixon, R. D., Best, T., Wilksch, S. R., Angelakis, S., Beatty, L. J., & Weber, N. (2016). Cognitive processing therapy for the treatment of acute stress disorder following sexual assault: A randomized effectiveness study. *Behaviour Change, 33*(4), 232–250. https://doi.org/10.1017/bec.2017.2

Norcross, J. C. (2002). *Psychotherapy relationships that work: Therapist contributions and responsiveness to patient needs*. Oxford University Press.

Norcross, J. C. (Ed.). (2011). *Psychotherapy relationships that work: Evidence-based responsiveness*. Oxford University Press.

O'Donohue, W., Carlson, G. C., Benuto, L. T., & Bennett, N. M. (2014). Examining the scientific validity of rape trauma syndrome. *Psychiatry, Psychology and Law, 21*(6), 858–876. https://doi.org/10.1080/13218719.2014.918067

Office for Victims of Crime. (2024). *History and development of SANE programs*. https://www.ovcttac.gov/saneguide/introduction/history-and-development-of-sane-programs/

Ogbe, E., Harmon, S., Van den Bergh, R., & Degomme, O. (2020). A systematic review of intimate partner violence interventions focused on improving social support and mental health outcomes of survivors. *PLOS ONE, 15*(6), e0235177. https://doi.org/10.1371/journal.pone.0235177

Pagelow, M. (1984). *Family violence*. Bloomsbury.

Pence, E., & Paymar, M. (1993). *Education groups for men who batter: The Duluth model*. Springer. https://doi.org/10.1891/9780826179913

Pence, E., & Shepard, M. (1999). Developing a coordinated community response: An introduction. In M. F. Shepard & E. L. Pence (Eds.), *Coordinating community responses to domestic violence: Lessons from the Duluth model* (pp. 3–23). Sage.

Platt, J. (1970). Hierarchical growth. *Bulletin of the Atomic Scientists, 26*(9), 2.

Prigogine, I., & Stengers, I. (2018). *Order out of chaos: Man's new dialogue with nature*. Verso Books.

Ramsay, J., Carter, Y., Davidson, L., Eldridge, S., Hegarty, K., Rivas, C., Taft, A., Warburton, A., Dunne, D., & Feder, G. (2009). PROTOCOL: Advocacy interventions to reduce or eliminate violence and promote the physical and psychosocial well-being of women who experience intimate partner abuse. *Campbell Systematic Reviews, 5*(1), 1–31. https://doi.org/10.1002/CL2.57

Rape, Abuse & Incest National Network. (2024a). *Effects of sexual violence*. https://rainn.org/effects-sexual-violence

Rape, Abuse & Incest National Network. (2024b). *RAINN's mission*. https://rainn.org/about-rainn

Rasmussen, H. N., Wrosch, C., Scheier, M. F., & Carver, C. S. (2006). Self-regulation processes and health: The importance of optimism and goal adjustment. *Journal of Personality, 74*(6), 1721–1748. https://doi.org/10.1111/j.1467-6494.2006.00426.x

Rescher, N. (1996). *Process metaphysics: An introduction to process philosophy.* SUNY Press.

Resick, P. A., Monson, C. M., & Chard, K. M. (2016). *Cognitive processing therapy for PTSD: A comprehensive manual.* Guilford Press.

Resick, P. A., Monson, C. M., & Chard, K. M. (2024). *Cognitive processing therapy for PTSD.* Guilford Press.

Reuters. (2024, April 26). *Harvey Weinstein: A timeline for sex crimes and overturned conviction.* https://www.reuters.com/world/us/rise-fall-movie-maker-harvey-weinstein-2024-04-25/

Richardson, V. E. (2010). The dual process model of coping with bereavement: A decade later. *Omega: Journal of Death and Dying, 61*(4), 269–271. https://doi.org/10.2190/OM.61.4.a

Rollè, L., Giardina, G., Caldarera, A. M., Gerino, E., & Brustia, P. (2018). When intimate partner violence meets same sex couples: A review of same sex intimate partner violence. *Frontiers in Psychology, 9,* 1506. https://doi.org/10.3389/fpsyg.2018.01506

Rollins, C., Glass, N. E., Perrin, N. A., Billhardt, K. A., Clough, A., Barnes, J., Hanson, G. C., & Bloom, T. L. (2012). Housing instability is as strong a predictor of poor health outcomes as level of danger in an abusive relationship: Findings from the SHARE study. *Journal of Interpersonal Violence, 27*(4), 623–643. https://doi.org/10.1177/0886260511423241

Rothenberg, B. (2003). We don't have time for social change: Cultural compromise and the battered woman syndrome. *Gender and Society, 17*(5), 771–787.

Rudd, M. D., Mandrusiak, M., & Joiner, T. E., Jr. (2006). The case against no-suicide contracts: The commitment to treatment statement as a practice alternative. *Journal of Clinical Psychology, 62*(2), 243–251. https://doi.org/10.1002/jclp.20227

Sardinha, L., Maheu-Giroux, M., Stöckl, H., Meyer, S. R., & García-Moreno, C. (2022). Global, regional, and national prevalence estimates of physical or sexual, or both, intimate partner violence against women in 2018. *The Lancet, 399*(10327), 803–813. https://doi.org/10.1016/S0140-6736(21)02664-7

Sarotte, M. E. (2014, November 6). How the fall of the Berlin Wall really happened. *The New York Times.* https://www.nytimes.com/2014/11/07/opinion/how-the-berlin-wall-really-fell.html

Scheper-Hughes, N. (1992). *Death without weeping: The violence of everyday life in Brazil.* University of California Press. https://doi.org/10.1525/9780520911567

Schonfeld, Z. (2024, January 27). E. Jean Carroll's legal fight against Trump: 10 key moments. *The Hill.* https://thehill.com/regulation/court-battles/4432789-e-jean-carroll-trump-legal-fight-key-moments/

Schorow, S. (2005). *The Cocoanut Grove fire*. Applewood Books.

Schuler, E. R., & Boals, A. (2016). Shattering world assumptions: A prospective view of the impact of adverse events on world assumptions. *Psychological Trauma: Theory, Research, Practice, and Policy, 8*(3), 259–266. https://doi.org/10.1037/tra0000073

Schut, H. (2010). Grief counselling efficacy: Have we learned enough? *Bereavement Care, 29*(1), 8–9. https://doi.org/10.1080/02682620903560817

Schut, M. S. H. (1999). The dual process model of coping with bereavement: Rationale and description. *Death Studies, 23*(3), 197–224. https://doi.org/10.1080/074811899201046

Segal, Z., Williams, J., & Teasdale, J. (2002). *Mindfulness-based cognitive therapy for depression: A new approach to relapse prevention*. Guilford Press.

Shapiro, F. (2012). EMDR therapy: An overview of current and future research. *European Review of Applied Psychology, 62*(4), 193–195. https://doi.org/10.1016/j.erap.2012.09.005

Shapiro, F. (2017). *Eye movement desensitization and reprocessing (EMDR) therapy: Basic principles, protocols, and procedures*. Guilford Press.

Sherman, L. W., & Berk, R. A. (1984). The specific deterrent effects of arrest for domestic assault. *American Sociological Review, 49*(2), 261–272. https://doi.org/10.2307/2095575

Shneidman, E. S. (1985, August 23–27). *Ten commonalities of suicide and some implications for public policy* [Paper presentation]. Annual Convention of the American Psychological Association, Los Angeles, CA, United States.

Shneidman, E. S. (1993). *Suicide as psychache: A clinical approach to self-destructive behavior*. Jason Aronson.

Shneidman, E. S., & Farberow, N. L. (1965). The Los Angeles suicide prevention center: A demonstration of public health feasibilies. *American Journal of Public Health and the Nation's Health, 55*(1), 21–26. https://doi.org/10.2105/AJPH.55.1.21

Smith, M. L., Glass, G. V., & Miller, T. I. (1980). *The benefits of psychotherapy*. The John Hopkins University Press.

Smith, S. G., Zhang, X., Basile, K. C., Merrick, M. T., Wang, J., Kresnow, M., & Chen, J. (2018, November 1). *The National Intimate Partner and Sexual Violence Survey: 2015 data brief—Updated release*. National Sexual Violence Resource Center. https://www.nsvrc.org/resource/2500/national-intimate-partner-and-sexual-violence-survey-2015-data-brief-updated-release

Snead, A. L., Bennett, V. E., & Babcock, J. C. (2018). Treatments that work for intimate partner violence: Beyond the Duluth model. In E. L. Jeglic & C. Calkins (Eds.), *New frontiers in offender treatment* (pp. 269–285). Springer. https://doi.org/10.1007/978-3-030-01030-0_14

Snyder, C. R., Michael, S. T., & Cheavens, J. S. (1999). Hope as a psychotherapeutic foundation of common factors, placebos, and expectancies. In M. A. Hubble, B. L. Duncan, & S. D. Miller (Eds.), *The heart and soul of change: What works in therapy* (pp. 179–200). American Psychological Association. https://doi.org/10.1037/11132-005

Soleymani, S., Britt, E., & Wallace-Bell, M. (2018). Motivational interviewing for enhancing engagement in intimate partner violence (IPV) treatment: A review of the literature. *Aggression and Violent Behavior, 40*, 119–127. https://doi.org/10.1016/j.avb.2018.05.005

Staw, B. M., Sandelands, L. E., & Dutton, J. E. (1981). Threat rigidity effects in organizational behavior: A multilevel analysis. *Administrative Science Quarterly, 26*(4), 501–524. https://doi.org/10.2307/2392337

Stroebe, M., Gergen, M. M., Gergen, K. J., & Stroebe, W. (1992). Broken hearts or broken bonds. Love and death in historical perspective. *American Psychologist, 47*(10), 1205–1212. https://doi.org/10.1037/0003-066X.47.10.1205

Stroebe, M. S., & Schut, H. (2001a). Meaning making in the dual process model of coping with bereavement. In R. A. Neimeyer (Ed.), *Meaning reconstruction & the experience of loss* (pp. 55–73). American Psychological Association. https://doi.org/10.1037/10397-003

Stroebe, M. S., & Schut, H. (2001b). Models of coping with bereavement: A review. In M. S. Stroebe, R. O. Hansson, W. Stroebe, & H. Schut (Eds.), *Handbook of bereavement research: Consequences, coping, and care* (pp. 375–403). American Psychological Association. https://doi.org/10.1037/10436-016

Stroebe, M. S., & Schut, H. (2008). The dual process model of coping with bereavement: Overview and update. *Grief Matters: The Australian Journal of Grief and Bereavement, 11*(1), 4–10.

Stroebe, M., & Schut, H. (2010). The dual process model of coping with bereavement: A decade on. *Omega: Journal of Death and Dying, 61*(4), 273–289. https://doi.org/10.2190/OM.61.4.b

Stroebe, M., & Schut, H. (2015). Family matters in bereavement: Toward an integrative intra-interpersonal coping model. *Perspectives on Psychological Science, 10*(6), 873–879. https://doi.org/10.1177/1745691615598517

Stroebe, M., & Schut, H. (2016). Overload: A missing link in the dual process model? *Omega: Journal of Death and Dying, 74*(1), 96–109. https://doi.org/10.1177/0030222816666540

Stroebe, M. S., Stroebe, W., & Hansson, R. O. (Eds.). (1993). *Handbook of bereavement: Theory, research, and intervention.* Cambridge University Press. https://doi.org/10.1017/CBO9780511664076

Stroebe, W., Schut, H., & Stroebe, M. S. (2005). Grief work, disclosure and counseling: Do they help the bereaved? *Clinical Psychology Review, 25*(4), 395–414. https://doi.org/10.1016/j.cpr.2005.01.004

Sullivan, C. M., Guerrero, M., Simmons, C., López-Zerón, G., Ayeni, O. O., Farero, A., Chiaramonte, D., & Sprecher, M. (2023). Impact of the domestic violence housing first model on survivors' safety and housing stability: 12-month findings. *Journal of Interpersonal Violence, 38*(5–6), 4790–4813. https://doi.org/10.1177/08862605221119520

Sullivan, C. M., López-Zerón, G., Farero, A., Ayeni, O. O., Simmons, C., Chiaramonte, D., Guerrero, M., Hamdan, N., & Sprecher, M. (2023). Impact of the domestic violence housing first model on survivors' safety and housing stability: Six-month findings. *Journal of Family Violence, 38*(3), 395–406. https://doi.org/10.1007/s10896-022-00381-x

Sullivan, C. M., Simmons, C., Guerrero, M., Farero, A., López-Zerón, G., Ayeni, O. O., Chiaramonte, D., Sprecher, M., & Fernandez, A. I. (2023). Domestic violence housing first model and association with survivors' housing stability, safety, and well-being over 2 years. *JAMA Network Open, 6*(6), e2320213. https://doi.org/10.1001/jamanetworkopen.2023.20213

Take Back the Night Foundation. (2023). *International history of TBTN*. https://takebackthenight.org/history/

Taku, K., Tedeschi, R. G., Shakespeare-Finch, J., Krosch, D., David, G., Kehl, D., Grunwald, S., Romeo, A., Di Tella, M., Kamibeppu, K., Soejima, T., Hiraki, K., Volgin, R., Dhakal, S., Zięba, M., Ramos, C., Nunes, R., Leal, I., Gouveia, P., . . . Calhoun, L. G. (2021). Posttraumatic growth (PTG) and posttraumatic depreciation (PTD) across ten countries: Global validation of the PTG-PTD theoretical model. *Personality and Individual Differences, 169*, 110222. https://doi.org/10.1016/j.paid.2020.110222

Tedeschi, R. G., & Calhoun, L. G. (1996). The Posttraumatic Growth Inventory: Measuring the positive legacy of trauma. *Journal of Traumatic Stress, 9*(3), 455–471. https://doi.org/10.1002/jts.2490090305

Tedeschi, R. G., & Calhoun, L. G. (2004a). A clinical approach to posttraumatic growth. *Positive Psychology in Practice*, 405–419.

Tedeschi, R. G., & Calhoun, L. G. (2004b). Posttraumatic growth: Conceptual foundations and empirical evidence. *Psychological Inquiry, 15*(1), 1–18. https://doi.org/10.1207/s15327965pli1501_01

Tedeschi, R. G., Calhoun, L. G., & Groleau, J. M. (2015). Clinical applications of posttraumatic growth. In S. Joseph (Ed.), *Positive psychology in practice: Promoting human flourishing in work, health, education, and everyday life* (pp. 503–518). Wiley. https://doi.org/10.1002/9781118996874.ch30

Trabold, N., McMahon, J., Alsobrooks, S., Whitney, S., & Mittal, M. (2020). A systematic review of intimate partner violence interventions: State of the field and implications for practitioners. *Trauma, Violence, & Abuse, 21*(2), 311–325. https://doi.org/10.1177/1524838018767934

Tryon, G. S., & Winograd, G. (2011). Goal consensus and collaboration. In J. C. Norcross (Ed.), *Psychotherapy relationships that work* (2nd ed., pp. 153–167). Oxford University Press. https://doi.org/10.1093/acprof:oso/9780199737208.003.0007

Ullman, S. E. (2023). *Talking about sexual assault: Society's response to survivors* (2nd ed.). American Psychological Association. https://doi.org/10.1037/0000360-000

Ulloa, E., Guzman, M. L., Salazar, M., & Cala, C. (2016). Posttraumatic growth and sexual violence: A literature review. *Journal of Aggression, Maltreatment & Trauma, 25*(3), 286–304. https://doi.org/10.1080/10926771.2015.1079286

U.S. Federal Bureau of Investigation. (2023, October 16). *FBI releases 2022 Crime in the Nation statistics*. https://www.fbi.gov/news/press-releases/fbi-releases-2022-crime-in-the-nation-statistics

van der Kolk, B. (2014). *The body keeps the score: Mind, brain and body in the transformation of trauma*. Penguin UK.

Violence Against Women Act of 1994, Pub. L. No. 103-322, 108 Stat. 1796 (1994). https://www.congress.gov/103/statute/STATUTE-108/STATUTE-108-Pg1796.pdf

Violence Against Women Act of 2005, Pub. L. No. 109-162, 119 Stat. 2960 (2005). https://www.congress.gov/bill/109th-congress/house-bill/3402

Violence Against Women Act Reauthorization Act of 2022, Pub. L. No. 117-103, 136 Stat. 49, Div. W of Consolidated Appropriations Act of 2022 (2022). https://www.congress.gov/bill/117th-congress/senate-bill/3623

Violence Against Women Reauthorization Act of 2013, Pub. L. No. 113-4, 127 Stat. 54 (2013). https://www.congress.gov/113/plaws/publ4/PLAW-113publ4.htm

Walker, L. E. (1999). Psychology and domestic violence around the world. *American Psychologist, 54*(1), 21–29. https://doi.org/10.1037/0003-066X.54.1.21

Walker, L. E. (2009). *The battered woman syndrome* (3rd ed.). Springer.

Walker, L. E. (2016). *The battered woman syndrome* (4th ed.). Springer.

Walker, L. E. A. (2006). Battered woman syndrome: Empirical findings. *Annals of the New York Academy of Sciences, 1087*(1), 142–157. https://doi.org/10.1196/annals.1385.023

Walters, M. L., Black, M. C., Basile, K. C., Breiding, M. J., Smith, S. G., Merrick, M. T., Stevens, M. R., & Chen, J. (2011). *The National Intimate Partner and Sexual Violence Survey (NISVS): 2010 summary report*. National Sexual Violence Resource Center. https://www.nsvrc.org/publications/NISVS-2010-summary-report

Wampold, B. E. (2001). *The great psychotherapy debate: Models, methods, and findings*. Lawrence Erlbaum.

Wampold, B. E., & Imel, Z. E. (2015). *The great psychotherapy debate: The evidence for what makes psychotherapy work* (2nd ed.). Routledge/Taylor & Francis Group.

Wampold, B. E., Mondin, G. W., Moody, M., Stich, F., Benson, K., & Ahn, H.-n. (1997). A meta-analysis of outcome studies comparing bona fide psychotherapies: Empirically, "all must have prizes." *Psychological Bulletin, 122*(3), 203–215. https://doi.org/10.1037/0033-2909.122.3.203

Warshaw, C., Rivera, E. A., & Sullivan, C. M. (2013). *A systematic review of trauma-focused interventions for domestic violence survivors*. National Center on Domestic Violence, Trauma, and Health. https://doi.org/10.1037/e566602013-001

Wasco, S. M. (2003). Conceptualizing the harm done by rape: Applications of trauma theory to experiences of sexual assault. *Trauma, Violence, & Abuse, 4*(4), 309–322. https://doi.org/10.1177/1524838003256560

Watters, E. (2011). *Crazy like us: The globalization of the Western mind.* Hachette.

Watzlawick, P., Bavelas, J. B., & Jackson, D. D. (1967). *Pragmatics of human communication: A study of interactional patterns, pathologies, and paradoxes.* W. W. Norton.

Watzlawick, P., Weakland, J. H., & Fisch, R. (1974). *Change: Principles of problem formation and problem resolution.* W. W. Norton.

Weisman, A. G., Rosales, G. A., Kymalainen, J. A., & Armesto, J. C. (2006). Ethnicity, expressed emotion, and schizophrenia patients' perceptions of their family members' criticism. *Journal of Nervous and Mental Disease, 194*(9), 644–649. https://doi.org/10.1097/01.nmd.0000235504.39284.f1

Weiss, T., & Berger, R. (2010). *Posttraumatic growth and culturally competent practice: Lessons learned from around the globe.* John Wiley & Sons. https://doi.org/10.1002/9781118270028

Whitehead, A. N. (1978). *Process and reality: An essay in cosmology.* The Free Press.

Wittouck, C., Van Autreve, S., De Jaegere, E., Portzky, G., & van Heeringen, K. (2011). The prevention and treatment of complicated grief: A meta-analysis. *Clinical Psychology Review, 31*(1), 69–78. https://doi.org/10.1016/j.cpr.2010.09.005

Wolfelt, A. (2007). *Companioning vs. treating: Beyond the medical model of bereavement caregiving.* Center for Loss and Life Transition, Massachusetts Funeral Directors Association.

Worden, J. W. (2002). *Grief counseling and grief therapy: A handbook for the mental health practitioner* (3rd ed.). Springer.

Worden, J. W. (2018). *Grief counseling and grief therapy: A handbook for the mental health practitioner* (5th ed.). Springer. https://doi.org/10.1891/9780826134752

Worden, J. W., & Winokuer, H. R. (2021). A task-based approach for counseling the bereaved. In *Grief and bereavement in contemporary society* (pp. 57–67). Routledge. https://doi.org/10.4324/9781003199762-7

World Health Organization. (2017). *International statistical classification of diseases and related health problems* (10th rev.). https://icd.who.int/

World Health Organization. (2021). *Suicide worldwide in 2019: Global health estimates.* https://www.who.int/publications/i/item/9789240026643

Wortman, C. B., & Silver, R. C. (1989). The myths of coping with loss. *Journal of Consulting and Clinical Psychology, 57*(3), 349–357. https://doi.org/10.1037/0022-006X.57.3.349

Wortman, C. B., Silver, R. C., & Kessler, R. C. (1993). The meaning of loss and adjustment to bereavement. In M. S. Stroebe, W. Stroebe, & R. O. Hansson (Eds.), *Handbook of bereavement: Theory, research, and intervention* (pp. 349–366). Cambridge University Press. https://doi.org/10.1017/CBO9780511664076.024

Zacharek, S., Dockterman, E., & Edwards, H. S. (2017, December 18). Person of the year 2017: The silence breakers. *Time.* https://time.com/time-person-of-the-year-2017-silence-breakers/

Zarling, A., Bannon, S., & Berta, M. (2019). Evaluation of acceptance and commitment therapy for domestic violence offenders. *Psychology of Violence, 9*(3), 257–266. https://doi.org/10.1037/vio0000097

Zarling, A., Bannon, S., Berta, M., & Russell, D. (2020). Acceptance and commitment therapy for individuals convicted of domestic violence: 5-year follow-up and time to reoffense. *Psychology of Violence, 10*(6), 667–675. https://doi.org/10.1037/vio0000292

Zarling, A., & Berta, M. (2017). An acceptance and commitment therapy approach for partner aggression. *Partner Abuse, 8*(1), 89–109. https://doi.org/10.1891/1946-6560.8.1.89

Zarling, A., Lawrence, E., & Marchman, J. (2015). A randomized controlled trial of acceptance and commitment therapy for aggressive behavior. *Journal of Consulting and Clinical Psychology, 83*(1), 199–212. https://doi.org/10.1037/a0037946

Zeeman, E. C. (1976). Catastrophe theory. *Scientific American, 234*(4), 65–83. https://doi.org/10.1038/scientificamerican0476-65

Zemeckis, R. (Director). (1994). *Forrest Gump* [Film]. Paramount Pictures.

Zoellner, T., & Maercker, A. (2006). Posttraumatic growth in clinical psychology: A critical review and introduction of a two component model. *Clinical Psychology Review, 26*(5), 626–653. https://doi.org/10.1016/j.cpr.2006.01.008

Zupancic, M., Huber, M., & Gilmore, B. (2016). *GBV and trauma-sensitive healthcare in Afghanistan: A baseline study*. Medica Afghanistan & Medica Mondiale. https://medicamondiale.org/fileadmin/redaktion/7_Service/1_Mediathek/1_Dokumente/2_English/Documentations_studies/Study-Medica-Afghanistan_GBV-Trauma_CR-Medica-Afghanistan_medica-mondiale.pdf

Index

A

ABC model structure, 62–63
Acceptance and commitment therapy
    (ACT), 171
Achieving Change Through Values-Based
    Behavior (ACTV), 171–174, 226
Acquiring suicidal capability, 109
ACT (acceptance and commitment
    therapy), 171
ACTV (Achieving Change Through Values-
    Based Behavior), 171–174, 226
Acute grief, 135
Adaptation of evidence-supported
    interventions, 61–62
Agility, at tipping points, 78
Aldwin, C. M., 93
Altmaier, E., 144
American Psychological Association (APA),
    42–43
Assumptions, 26–27
    about the world, 92–94
    at crisis points, 218
    in traditional views of crisis, 17–20
Attractors
    butterfly, 30
    crisis, 33, 47–48, 189
    defined, 33
    point, 30
    vortex of, 32
Avoidance symptoms, in PTSD, 82

B

Barner, J. R., 164–166
Basile, K. C., 190

Bateson, Gregory, 86
Battered woman cycle model, 176
Battered woman's syndrome, 176–178
Batterers groups, 169–171
B-CPT (brief cognitive processing
    therapy), 205
Being there, in grief and mourning,
    144–145
Beneficent perpetrators, 177
Benish, S. G., 90
Bereavement, 135. *See also* Grief and
    mourning
Berger, R., 94
Berlin Wall, 7–8, 19, 35
Berta, M., 172
Berwick, D. M., 5
Biological model of systems, 18
The Body Keeps the Score (van der Kolk),
    85–86
Bonanno, G. A., 140
Both–and phenomenon, 94
Bowlby, John, 136
Brazil, angel babies in, 134
Break/recess (step 4), 65
Brewin, C. R., 84–85
Brief cognitive processing therapy
    (B-CPT), 205
Brief therapy
    process of change model in. *See* Process
        of change model of crisis and crisis
        intervention
    for sexual assault, 205
    traditional, 3
Briggs, J., 23, 28, 29, 33

Bringing in the Bystander, 200
Bryan, C. J., 109–110
Buckley, Walter, 18
Budman, S. H., 43–44, 229
Building a Therapeutic Alliance With the Suicidal Patient (Michel & Jobes), 110, 115
Burgess, A. W., 202
Burke, Tarana, 196
Burnout, combating, 221–223
Butterfly attractors, 30
Butterfly effect, 19
Bystander effect, 200
Bystander intervention, with sexual assault, 200

C

Caldwell, J. E., 161
Calhoun, L. G., 91–93, 95, 207
Campbell, R., 198, 199
CAMS (clinical assessment and management of suicide), 115, 118
Cann, A., 93
Caplan, Gerald, 16, 17, 42, 43
Carney, M. M., 164–166
Carroll, E. Jean, 185, 196–197
Carver, C. S., 93
Catastrophe, 13, 34–35
Catastrophe theory, 34–37
CBT. *See* Cognitive behavior therapy
Change. *See also* Shifts
    assumptions about, 19
    continual, 218
    creative, 26
    importance of rapid intervention for, 43
    models of, 19, 20
    and stability, 24–25
    that initiate crises, 35
    transformational, 13, 14, 218, 220
    unexpected, perception of, 219–220
Chaos, 13
    defined, 16
    and flow, 29–31
    making sense of chaotic world, 23–24
    and process, 28–29
Chaos (Gleick), 23, 28, 29
Chaos theory, 16, 28, 33
Chiles, J. A., 105–107, 109–112, 115, 116, 120–123
Clark, D. M., 84

Client variables, 66, 67. *See also specific types of crises*
Clinical assessment and management of suicide (CAMS), 115, 118
Cocoanut Grove nightclub fire, 15, 16, 135
Cognitions, negative alterations in, 82
Cognitive behavior therapy (CBT)
    for intimate partner violence, 167–169, 173
    for sexual assault, 205, 206
    in suicide intervention, 121
Cognitive fusion and diffusion, 172
Cognitive processing therapy (CPT), 88
Cognitive theories, posttraumatic stress disorder and, 84–85
Cognitive trauma therapy for battered women (CTT-BW), 168
Commitment-to-treatment contracts, 113
Compassion fatigue, 127, 221–223
Complex grieving, 147, 225
Complicated grief, 140, 225
Complicated grief disorder, 141
Condino, V., 170
Consensual problem formation and goal setting (step 3), 64–65
Constructivist theories, PTSD and, 85
Context, 31–32. *See also* Cultural context
    importance of, 20
    intimate partner violence in, 158–162
    of the observer, 36
    positive, for disclosure, 96
    in process of change, 58, 66–68
    of sexual assault, 188–192
    in suicide intervention, 118–119
Continual change, 218
Contracts
    commitment-to-treatment, 113
    no-suicide, 111–114
    therapy, 66–68
Cost of caring, 223
Counterintuitive habits, 24–25
Counterintuitive solutions to crises, 3–7, 220
CPT (cognitive processing therapy), 88
Creative change, 26–27
Crisis(—es), 3–7. *See also specific types of crises*
    assumptions about, 19–20
    counterintuitive or illogical reactions to, 3–7
    crisis attractors, 33, 47–48, 189
    individual, 17

key concepts related to, 45–51
as mirror image of crisis intervention, 41–42
problem-generated systems around, 49
problem patterns in, 50–51
process-based view of, 51–54. *See also* Process of change (process-based view) of crises
reframing, 8
relative nature of, 7–8, 36–37
as solution-generated problems, 48–49
as threats to presumed stability, 218
as tipping points, 217
traditional definition of, 17–19
trigger points of, 45–47
varying uses of term, vii–viii
vicious and virtuous cycles in, 3, 6–7
window of opportunity for rapid intervention, 42–43
Crisis attractors, 33, 47–48, 189
Crisis intervention. *See also specific types of crises*
adapting evidence-supported interventions, 61–62
as mirror image of crisis, 41–42
pattern change as target of, 37
process of change model in. *See* Process of change model of crisis and crisis intervention
process view of, 41–42
rapid, 42–45
successful, 228
traditional, 3, 6
views affecting, 51–54. *See also* Process of change (process-based view) of crisis intervention
CTT-BW (cognitive trauma therapy for battered women), 168
Cubic model of suicide, 108
Cultural context, 66, 67
of grief and mourning, 138–139
of intimate partner violence, 158–162
of sexual assault, 186–188, 190–192, 199–201
in suicide intervention, 116–117
Cultural humility, 204
Cultural-level interventions
in intimate partner violence, 162–165, 182–183
with sexual assault, 192–201
Cultural traditions, 48
Culture wars movement, 194–195

Currier, J. M., 139–140, 148
Cycle of violence perspective, 176–177

D

Danger, perceiving, 19
DBT. *See* Dialectical behavior therapy
Death and dying, 131–135. *See also* Grief and mourning; Suicide
Delayed grief, 135
Deliberative rumination, 93
Depression models of grief, 136
de Shazer, S., 5
Developmental life crises, 46
defined, 46
grief and mourning as, 225–226
origin of trigger points in, 45, 46
Dialectical behavior therapy (DBT), 113, 115, 120
Direct clinical level interventions
for intimate partner violence, 158, 165–176, 182
for sexual assault, 201–208
Disclosure
in positive context, 96
of sexual assault, 196
Distorted grief reactions, 135–136
Distress, validating, 119
Dodge, Wag, 5
Doka, K. J., 147–148
Domestic violence, 158. *See also* Intimate partner violence (IPV)
Domestic Violence Housing First, 167
Domestic violence shelter movement, 163–164
DPM (dual process model), 145–148
Dual process model (DPM), 145–148
Duluth model, 164–165, 167, 168, 173
Durkheim, Emile, 108
Dworkin, E. R., 196

E

Eckhardt, C. I., 161, 168–169
Ehlers, A., 84
EMDR. *See* Eye movement desensitization and reprocessing
Emotional avoidance, 95
Endemic life crises, 47
defined, 47
intimate partner violence as, 158, 183, 226–227

origin of trigger points in, 45, 47
sexual assault and rape as, 186–192,
   227–228
Episodes of care model, 52
Equality wheel, 164–165
Equifinality, 47
Equilibrium, 18
Evidence-supported interventions, 61–62
Experiential avoidance, 172
Exposure-based approaches, for PTSD,
   88–89, 224
Eye movement desensitization and
   reprocessing (EMDR)
for PTSD, 88
for sexual assault, 205, 206

F

Failed belongingness, 109
Farberow, Norman, 108
Feedback, in systemic causation, 22
Feminist movement, 192–193
Figley, C. R., 223
Figley, K. R., 223
Fiore, J., 146
First-order solutions, 26, 106
First-wave feminism, 192
Fisch, R., 26
Fischer, P., 200
Fit, 45
in grief and mourning, 143, 148
in intimate partner violence
   interventions, 170–171
in process of change model, 66
in sexual assault interventions, 206
in trauma intervention, 97
Fitting shift, in grief and mourning, 143
Flexibility, 44–45
in grief and mourning intervention,
   143, 148
in intimate partner violence
   interventions, 170–171
psychological, 173
in sexual assault interventions, 206
in trauma intervention, 97
Flow, chaos and, 29–31
Focusing on the relationship, in grief and
   mourning, 144
Forrest Gump (movie), 35–36
Fourth-wave feminism, 192
Fractals, 31, 34
Frank, Jerome, 68–69

Fraser, J. S., 5, 8, 224
Freud, S., 136

G

Gender focus, in intimate partner violence,
   160–163, 176, 226
Generic intervention options
in process-based view of crisis
   intervention, 68–72
with suicide, 118–124
Generic problem definitions, 66
Generic response patterns, 50, 51
formed around vicious cycles, 217
in grief and mourning, 137
in intimate partner violence, 175
rape trauma syndrome as, 202–204
with sexual assault, 204–205
Gergen, Kenneth, 32
Ghana, celebrations of death in, 134
Gilliland, B. E., 17, 114, 138
Gladwell, Malcolm, 16, 23
Gleick, James, 23, 29
Goals
in Achieving Change Through Values-
   Based Behavior approach, 171–174
for crisis resolution, 60
for intimate partner violence
   interventions, 174–175, 182–183
of process of change perspective, 66,
   174–175, 220
setting, 64–65
Goerner, S., 47
Gore, Al, vii
Gradualism, 35
Graham, D. L., 176–177
Grant, A., 23, 25
Grant, Adam, 23–24
Grief (term), 135
Grief and mourning, 131–155
applying process of change model to,
   149–155
being there in, 144–145
as developmental crisis, 225–226
dual process model with, 145–148
growing beyond, 148–149
history of grief models, 135–139
intervening in, 139–142
making meaning of loss with, 148
process of change approach to, 142–144
Grief work, 135
Groleau, J. M., 93

Growth
    beyond grief and mourning, 148–149
    posttraumatic. *See* Posttraumatic growth
        (PTG)
Gurman, A. S., 43–44, 229

H

Hackett, S., 168
Hayes, Steven, 171
Hazardous intersections, viii, 118
Helping to Overcome PTSD Through
    Empowerment (HOPE), 168
Heraclitus, 27–30, 33
History
    of grief models, 135–139
    within occurrence of crises, 58
    of process view, 27–28
Holmstrom, L. L., 202
Homeostasis, 18
Hope, 69, 121
HOPE (Helping to Overcome PTSD
    Through Empowerment), 168
Hoppe, S. J., 165
"How a Misunderstanding About Chinese
    Characters Has Led Many Astray"
    (Mair), vii
"How the Fall of the Berlin Wall Really
    Happened" (Sarotte), 7
Humphrey, K. M., 147
Hyperarousal, in PTSD, 82

I

Ideas, process-based systems and, 219
Imel, Z. E., 90, 173
Incidental life crises, 46
    defined, 46
    origin of trigger points in, 45, 46
    suicide as, 225
Individual crisis, 17
Information gathering (step 2), 64
Information processing theory, PTSD and,
    84
International Women's Day (IWD), 195–196
Interpersonal theory of suicide, 109,
    116–118, 120, 122
Intervening process, influence of, 47
Intimate partner violence (IPV), 157–184
    Achieving Change Through Values-Based
        Behavior for, 171–174
    batterers groups for, 169–171

    changing laws about, 162–163
    cognitive behavior therapy for,
        167–169
    in context, 158–162
    cultural-level interventions in,
        162–165
    direct clinical level interventions in,
        165–174
    Duluth model with, 164–165
    as endemic crisis, 158, 226–227
    incidence of, 159–160
    mindfulness skills for, 173–174
    moving from gender focus on to power
        and control, 161–162
    and pattern of battered woman's
        syndrome, 176–178
    perpetrator interventions for, 169–174
    process of change model for, 178–181,
        183–184
    reversing patterns in, 182–183
    and shelter movement, 163–164
    social advocacy for, 167
    tipping points with, 174–178
    women's groups for, 166–167
Intrusive rumination, 93
Intuitive grieving, 147–148
IPV. *See* Intimate partner violence
It's a Wonderful Life (movie), 6, 19
IWD (International Women's Day),
    195–196

J

James, R. K., 17, 114, 138
Janoff-Bulman, R., 95
Ji (jei), 77–78, 208, 218
Jobes, D. A., 105, 107, 110, 115, 118, 120,
    122
Joiner, T. E., 109, 115–117
Joseph, S., 149
"Just world" myth, 85

K

Kahneman, Daniel, 23–25, 106, 218
Kennedy, A. C., 205
Kennedy, John F., vii
Kessler, R. C., 82–83
Kick points, in process of change, 58
Know My Name (Miller), 197
Koss, M. P., 189, 204
Kübler-Ross, Elisabeth, 136–138

L

Lang, P. J., 84
Lao Tzu, 27–29, 33
Learned helplessness, 176
Learning theory, PTSD and, 83–84
Levy, R., 197
Life, assumptions about, 92–93
Lilienfeld, S. O., 140
Limit cycles, 30
Lindemann, Erich, 16, 17, 135–136
Linehan, Marsha, 113, 115, 120
Linley, P. A., 149
Lomax, J., 206
Loss
  grieving and mourning. *See* Grief and
    mourning
  making meaning of, 148
  terms associated with, 135
Loss-oriented coping mechanisms, 144
Ludick, M., 223

M

Maercker, A., 94–96
Maier, S. F., 176
Mair, Victor H., vii
Making meaning of loss, 148
Martin, P. Y., 198
Martin, T. L., 147–148
Mastery by avoidance, 172, 205
Mattsson, M., 197
MBCBT (mindfulness-based cognitive
  behavior therapy), 121, 122
McDonagh, A., 89
McLeod, D. A., 161
Meaning
  making meaning of loss, 148
  search for, following trauma, 93–94
Mechanical systems, 18
The Men's Program, 200
Mental illness, outdated notions of, 110
Messing, J. T., 163, 178
#MeToo movement, 189, 196–197
Meyrick, J., 206
Michael, T., 95
Michel, K. E., 105, 107, 110, 115, 120
Micklitz, H. M., 161
Milano, Alyssa, 196
Miles, L. W., 206
Miller, Chanel, 186, 197
Miller, M. C., 112–113

Mindfulness-based cognitive behavior
  therapy (MBCBT), 121, 122
Mindfulness skills
  in ACTV, 172–173
  for intimate partner violence, 173–174
Mood, negative alterations in, 82
Morbid grief reactions, 135
Mourning, 135. *See also* Grief and
  mourning
Mourning and Melancholia (Freud), 136
Mowrer, O. H., 83–84
Mujal, G. N., 200
Multideterminism, 142
Multifinality, 47, 142
Murphy-Oikonen, J., 191

N

National Council of Mental Wellbeing, 42
Negative alterations in cognitions and
  mood, in PTSD, 82
Negative feedback, 22
Negative repeated rumination, 94
Neimeyer, R. A., 93, 139–140, 142, 148
Network of others involved, in process of
  change, 60
Nixon, R. D., 206
Normal grief, 135, 136
Normalizing
  as generic intervention option, 69–70
  in suicide interventions, 121
No-suicide contracts, problem with,
  111–114

O

O'Donohue, W., 203
Office on Violence Against Women, 162,
  193
Ogbe, E., 167
On Death and Dying (Kübler-Ross), 136
One-down position, 70
Opportunity, perceiving, 19
Organismic systems, 18
Overload, in lives of the bereaved,
  146–147

P

Pagelow, M., 177
Panic attacks, 8

Paradox, 26–27
  defined, 26
  of effective interventions for sexual
      assaults, 205
Patriarchy, 160, 188
Patterns
  around types of crises, 48
  from chaos, 35
  fractal, 34
  problem, 50–51. *See also* Problem patterns
  of process, 33
  shifts and reversals in, 60–61, 66, 166,
      175, 182
  successful shifts in, 62
  of vicious cycles, 36–37. *See also* Vicious
      cycles
PCT (present-centered therapy), 88–91
PE. *See* Prolonged exposure
Peat, F. D., 23, 28, 29, 33
Perceived burdensomeness, 109
Perpetrator interventions, with intimate
      partner violence, 169–174
Persistent complex bereavement disorder,
      141
Phase models of grief, 137–139
Phase space, 31
Physiologically based theories, PTSD and,
      85–86
Point attractors, 30
Positioning
  as generic intervention option, 71
  in suicide interventions, 119
Positive feedback, 22
Posttraumatic growth (PTG), 79, 91–96
  as alternative to PTSD view, 91–92
  and assumptions of life and the world,
      92–93
  and disclosure in positive context, 96
  with grief and mourning, 148–149
  in positively resolving crises and
      trauma, 94–96
  in searching for meaning, 93–94
  from sexual assault, 206–208
Posttraumatic stress disorder (PTSD), 79,
      81–91
  cognitive theories' views of, 84–85
  constructivist theories' views of, 85
  definitions of, 81
  example of, 79–81
  exposure-based approaches to, 88–89
  information processing theory view of,
      84

learning theory view of, 83–84
  physiologically based theories of, 85–86
  posttraumatic growth as alternative
      view to, 91–92
  present-centered therapy for, 89–91
  prevalence of, 82–83
  with sexual violence, 203
  symptoms of, 81–82
  treatments that work for, 88
  vicious cycles of, 86–88
Power and control wheel, 164, 166
Power positions, 177
Predictability, quest for, 22–23
Predicting
  as generic intervention option, 71–72
  in suicide interventions, 123–124
Predicting suicide, 106–108
Prescribing
  as generic intervention option, 71
  in suicide interventions, 121–123
Present-centered therapy (PCT), 88–91
Problem-generated systems, 218
  around crises, 49
  solution-generated problems within, 143
Problem-generating solution patterns, 87.
      See also Vicious cycles
Problem patterns, 50–51
  in intimate partner violence, 182–183
  rape trauma syndrome as, 202–204
Problem solving
  in approach to suicide, 113–114
  common premises, assumptions, and
      rules in, 26
Problem solving and interventions
      (step 5), 65
Process
  and chaos, 28–29
  patterns of, 33
Process and Reality (Whitehead), 27
PROCESS model, 224
Process of change model of crisis and crisis
      intervention, 3–7, 21–39
  break/recess (step 4) in, 65
  and catastrophe theory, 34–37
  and chaos and flow, 29–31
  consensual problem formation and goal
      setting (step 3) in, 64–65
  context in, 31–32, 66–68
  contracting in, 66–68
  crisis attractors in, 33
  defined, 58
  essence of, 13

and feedback in systemic causation, 22
and fractals, 34
general interventions of, 221
generic options vs., 68–72
with grief and mourning, 149–155,
    225–226
history of process view, 27–28
information gathering (step 2) in, 64
intervention process in, 62–68. *See also*
    specific types of crises
with intimate partner violence, 178–181,
    183–184, 226–227
key elements of, 10, 72–73
making sense of chaotic world in, 23–24
paradox and creative change in, 26–27
principles of, 220
problem solving and interventions
    (step 5) in, 65
process and chaos in, 28–29
and quest for stable, predictable world,
    22–23
relationship establishment (step 1) in,
    63–64
with sexual assault, 208–216, 227–228
stability and change in, 24–25
steps in, 62–66, 220
for suicide, 114–118, 124–129, 225
summary and closure (step 6) in, 65
summary of, 37–39
and threat rigidity hypothesis, 25–26
traditional crisis intervention vs., 20
for trauma, 96–103, 224–225
Process of change (process-based view) of
    crises, 41–54
key crisis concepts in, 45–51
and key elements of all rapid
    intervention, 43–45
model for. *See* Process of change model
    of crisis and crisis intervention
that affect crisis interventions, 51–54
as window of opportunity for rapid
    intervention, 42–43
Process of change (process-based view) of
    crisis intervention, 41–42, 55–73
examples of, 55–62
generic options in, 68–72
model for, 62–68. *See also* Process of
    change model of crisis and crisis
    intervention
Process of change (process-based)
    perspective, 20
adapting evidence-supported
    interventions in, 61–62

advantages of, 41–42
context and history in, 58
of crises, 6–7, 51–54. *See also* Process of
    change (process-based view) of crises
crises in, 219–220
goals for crisis resolution in, 60
in grief disruption, 142–144
history of, 27–28, 58
with intimate partner violence, 174–178
kick points, triggers, or shifts in, 58
network of others involved in, 60
pattern shifts and reversals in, 60–61
pattern-shift successes in, 62
reaction targeting resolution in, 59
response to solution attempts in, 59–60
traditional crisis intervention vs., 20.
    See also Process of change (process-
    based view) of crisis intervention
views, values, strengths, and resources
    in, 61
Process philosophy, 27–28
Process view of the world, history of,
    27–28
Prock, K. A., 205
Prolonged exposure (PE)
for PTSD, 88
for sexual assault, 205, 206
Psychache, 108–105
Psychological flexibility, 173
PTG. *See* Posttraumatic growth
PTSD. *See* Posttraumatic stress disorder

Q

Quest for stable, predictable world, 22–23
Quickness, at tipping points, 78

R

Radical feminism, 192
Radical listening, 204
RAINN (Rape, Abuse & Incest National
    Network), 200
Rape. *See also* Sexual assault
definitions of, 189–190
as endemic crisis, 188–192
incidence of, 190, 195
secondary victimization with, 197–198
underreporting of, 190–192, 195–196
Rape, Abuse & Incest National Network
    (RAINN), 200
Rape crisis centers, 192–193, 201

Rape trauma syndrome (RTS), 201–204
Rapid intervention
    as first choice for practice, 42, 229
    key elements of, 43–45
    window of opportunity for, 42–43
Rationales, 66, 68–69
Reexperiencing, in PTSD, 81–82
Reframing, 8
    as generic intervention option, 68, 69
    with sexual assault, 205, 206
    in suicide interventions, 119–121
Relationship establishment (step 1), 63–64
Relative nature of crises, 7–8
Rescher, Nicholas, 27–28
Resick, P. A., 85
Resourcefulness, at tipping points, 78
Resources, in process of change, 61
Restoration-oriented coping mechanisms, 144
Restraining
    as generic intervention option, 70–71
    in suicide interventions, 119
Reversals, pattern, 60–61, 166, 175, 182
Risk management stance, 218
Risk-oriented assessments of suicide, treatment-oriented assessments vs., 110–112
Risky shifts, 43
Rollè, L., 160
RTS (rape trauma syndrome), 201–204
Rudd, M. D., 113
Rumination, 93–95

S

Safe havens, 43
SANE (Sexual Assault Nurse Examiners), 197–199
Sardinha, L., 160
Sarotte, M. E., 7
Scheier, M. F., 93
Schumacher, J. A., 196
Schut, H., 140, 145–147
SCRIPT protocol, 122–123
Search for meaning, following trauma, 93–94
Secondary trauma, combating, 221, 222
Secondary victimization, with sexual assault and rape, 190–191, 197–198
Second-order change, 26
    with sexual assault, 205
    in suicide, 106

Second-wave feminism, 192
Seligman, M. E., 176
Sexual assault, 185–216
    applying process of change model with, 208–216
    battle to change cultural context of, 199–201
    bystander intervention with, 200
    context of, 188–192
    crisis attractors in, 189
    cultural-level interventions with, 192–201
    and culture wars movement, 194–195
    definitions of, 189–190
    direct clinical level interventions for, 201–208
    effective interventions with survivors of, 204–208
    as endemic crisis, 227–228
    incidence of, 190–192
    and International Women's Day, 195–196
    and #MeToo movement, 196–197
    posttraumatic growth from, 206–208
    rape crisis centers, 192–193, 201
    rape trauma syndrome as generic pattern, 202–204
    Sexual Assault Nurse Examiners, 197–199
    tipping points for, 189
    underreporting of, 190–192
    Violence Against Women Act of 1994, 193–195
Sexual Assault Nurse Examiners (SANE), 197–199
Shattered assumption theory, 92–93
Shelter movement, 163–164
Shi, 77–78
Shifts
    in grief and mourning, 143
    in patterns, 60–61, 66, 166, 175, 182
    in process of change, 58
    risky, 43
    successful, 62
Shneidman, Edwin, 108
Snead, A. L., 159, 171
Social advocacy, for intimate partner violence, 167
Social systems, 18, 47–48
Sociocultural process-based systems, 18–19
Soleymani, S., 170, 171

Solution attempts, response to, 59–60
Solution-generated problems, 218
   crises as, 41, 48–49
   in intimate partner violence, 175
   within potentially problem-generated
      systems, 143
Specific client problem definition, 66
Specific response patterns, 50–51
Stability
   assumptions about, 19, 20
   and change, 24–25
   as the norm, 218
   quest for, 22–23
Stage models of grief, 136–139
Staw, B. M., 25
Stockholm syndrome, 176–177
Strengths, in process of change, 61
Stress inoculation training, 88
Stroebe, M. S., 135, 145–147
Stroebe, W., 140
Strosahl, K. D., 105–107, 109–112, 115,
      116, 120–123
Suicide, 105–129
   attending to context approach for,
      118–119
   contextualizing and validating distress
      approach with, 119
   cultural views of, 32n
   generic interventions in approaches to
      tipping points for, 118–124
   helpline for, 107
   normalizing with, 121
   as not a "thing in itself," 109–110
   offering rationales and reframing
      approach with, 119–121
   positioning and restraining with, 119
   as potential incidental crisis, 225
   predicting, 106–108
   predicting approach with, 123–124
   prescribing with, 121–123
   and problem with no-suicide contracts,
      111–114
   process of change model case example
      for, 124–129
   and promising pathways to positive
      intersections, 114–118
   psychache and tipping points for,
      108–105
   risk-oriented vs. treatment-oriented
      assessments of, 110–112
   statistics on, 107
   Three I's of, 109, 110

Summary and closure (step 6), 65
Survivor (term), 190, 193
Survivor analysis, 170
Symptom prescriptions, in suicide
      intervention, 122
System 1, 24–25, 106, 218
System 2, 24–25, 106, 218
Systemic causation, feedback in, 22
Systems
   crises in context of, 17–18
   levels of, 18–19
   problem-generated, 49
   social, 18, 47–48

T

Take Back the Night marches, 195
Taku, K., 96
Task models of grief, 137–139
Tedeschi, R. G., 91–93, 95, 207
Therapeutic alliance, 66–68. *See also
      specific types of crises*
Therapist variables, 66, 67. *See also specific
      types of crises*
Therapy contract, 66–68
Think Again (Grant), 23–24
Thinking, Fast and Slow (Kahneman), 23–24
Third-wave feminism, 192
Threat rigidity hypothesis, 25–26, 106, 218
Three I's, 109, 110, 225
Time Magazine, 196, 201
The Tipping Point (Gladwell), 16, 23
Tipping points, 77–78, 217–223
   as catastrophes, 36
   from clients' vs. practitioners' side, 41
   crises as, 217
   defined, viii, 16
   interpretations of, 4
   with intimate partner violence, 174–178
   for sexual assault, 189
   for suicide, 105, 107–109
   for vicious cycles, 219
Trabold, N., 167, 168
Traditional brief therapy, 3
Traditional crisis intervention, 3, 6, 15–20
   and common understanding/
      experiences of world, 22–23
   "defining" crisis in, 17–19
   focus on stability in, 218
   limitations of, 77
   misguided assumptions in, 17–18
   problems with, 19–20

process of change perspective vs., 20
system levels in, 18–19
Transformational change
in process of change perspective, 13, 14
supporting virtuous cycles toward, 218
virtuous cycles in, 220
Trauma, 79–103. *See also specific types of trauma*
as common aspect across crises, 224–225
example of, 79–81
phases of recovery from, 83
and posttraumatic growth, 91–96. *See also* Posttraumatic growth (PTG)
process of change approach to, 96–103
and PTSD, 81–91. *See also* Posttraumatic stress disorder (PTSD)
vicious cycles following, 87
Treatment-oriented assessments of suicide, risk-oriented assessments vs., 110–112
Trigger points
of crises, 45–47, 217
in process of change, 58
for vicious cycles, 219
Trump, Donald, 185, 196–197
Turbulence, 29, 30–31, 36
Turbulent Mirror (Briggs & Peat), 29
Turner, Brock, 186, 197, 200
Tversky, Amos, 24

U

Ullman, S. E., 189, 192
Ulloa, E., 207–208
Underserved populations, 194
Unifying Effective Psychotherapies (Fraser), 224

V

Validating distress, in suicide intervention, 119
Values
in Achieving Change Through Values-Based Behavior approach, 171–174
in process of change, 61
Van der Kolk, Bessel, 85–86
VAWA. *See* Violence Against Women Act of 1994; Violence Against Women Reauthorization Act of 2022
Vicious cycles, 3, 6–7, 30
as escalation of well-meaning solution attempts, 41

generic patterns formed by, 217
in grief and mourning, 143
in intimate partner violence, 167
patterns of, 36–37
in posttraumatic stress disorder, 86–88
as solution-generated problems, 48–49
in systems in crisis, 218
triggers or tipping points for, 219
Victims (term), 190
Vietnam, death day in, 134
Views, in process of change, 61
Violence Against Women Act of 1994 (VAWA), 162, 163, 193–195
Violence Against Women Reauthorization Act of 2022 (VAWA), 194–195
Virtuous cycles, 3, 30
in grief and mourning, 143
in sexual assault, 189
supporting, 218
of transformation, 220

W

Walker, Lenore, 176–178
Walters, M. L., 159–160
Wampold, B. E., 173
Warshaw, C., 159
Wasco, S. M., 203–204
Watzlawick, P., 26
Weakland, J. H., 26
Wei ji (jei), vii, viii, 208, 218
Weinstein, Harvey, 185–186, 196
Weiss, T., 94
Whitehead, A. N., 28
Whitehead, Alfred North, 27
Wife battering, 158. *See also* Intimate partner violence (IPV)
Window of opportunity, viii
in crises, 217
for disclosure of sexual assault, 196
for rapid intervention, 42–43
Wisdom, at tipping points, 78
Wittouck, C., 140
Wolfelt, A., 138–139
Women's groups, 166–167
Wortman, C. B., 137

Z

Zarling, A., 170, 172, 173
Zeeman, E. C., 36
Zoellner, T., 94–96

About the Author

J. Scott Fraser, PhD, is a clinical psychologist with nearly 40 years of clinical practice, supervision, training, and academic teaching experience. He has served as director of internship training, associate dean, director of clinical training, and professor of clinical psychology in the doctoral program at the School of Professional Psychology at the Wright State University in Dayton, Ohio. Before that, he was director of a crisis/brief therapy center in a large general hospital setting for 14 years. He has published many papers and books, including *Unifying Effective Psychotherapies: Tracing the Process of Change*, and the video *The Process of Change in Integrative Psychotherapy*, which uses the process model described in this book.